VOLUME ONE HUNDRED AND TWENTY NINE

INTERNATIONAL REVIEW OF NEUROBIOLOGY

Imaging the Addicted Brain

INTERNATIONAL REVIEW OF NEUROBIOLOGY

VOLUME 129

VOLUME ONE HUNDRED AND TWENTY NINE

INTERNATIONAL REVIEW OF NEUROBIOLOGY

Imaging the Addicted Brain

Edited by

NATALIE M. ZAHR
Neuroscience Program,
SRI International,
Menlo Park, CA, United States

Psychiatry & Behavioral Sciences,
Stanford University School of Medicine,
Stanford, CA, United States

ERIC T. PETERSON
Neuroscience Program,
SRI International,
Menlo Park, CA, United States

ELSEVIER

AMSTERDAM • BOSTON • HEIDELBERG • LONDON
NEW YORK • OXFORD • PARIS • SAN DIEGO
SAN FRANCISCO • SINGAPORE • SYDNEY • TOKYO
Academic Press is an imprint of Elsevier

AP

Academic Press is an imprint of Elsevier
50 Hampshire Street, 5th Floor, Cambridge, MA 02139, United States
525 B Street, Suite 1800, San Diego, CA 92101-4495, United States
The Boulevard, Langford Lane, Kidlington, Oxford OX5 1GB, United Kingdom
125 London Wall, London, EC2Y 5AS, United Kingdom

First edition 2016

Notices
Knowledge and best practice in this field are constantly changing. As new research and experience broaden our understanding, changes in research methods, professional practices, or medical treatment may become necessary.

Practitioners and researchers must always rely on their own experience and knowledge in evaluating and using any information, methods, compounds, or experiments described herein. In using such information or methods they should be mindful of their own safety and the safety of others, including parties for whom they have a professional responsibility.

To the fullest extent of the law, neither the Publisher nor the authors, contributors, or editors, assume any liability for any injury and/or damage to persons or property as a matter of products liability, negligence or otherwise, or from any use or operation of any methods, products, instructions, or ideas contained in the material herein.

ISBN: 978-0-12-803914-4
ISSN: 0074-7742

For information on all Academic Press publications visit our website at https://www.elsevier.com/

Publisher: Zoe Kruze
Acquisition Editor: Kirsten Shankland
Editorial Project Manager: Hannah Colford
Production Project Manager: Surya Narayanan Jayachandran
Cover Designer: Mathew Limbert

Typeset by SPi Global, India

CONTENTS

CONTRIBUTORS

I.M. Balodis
Yale University, New Haven, CT, United States

T. Brumback
University of California, San Diego, La Jolla; VA San Diego Healthcare System, San Diego, CA, United States

N. Castro
University of California, San Diego, La Jolla, CA, United States

S. Chanraud
EPHE, PSL Research University, Bordeaux, France

D.B. de Araujo
Brain Institute/Hospital Universitario Onofre Lopes, UFRN, Natal, Brazil

L.T. Dowdle
Medical University of South Carolina, Charleston, SC, United States

M. Dupuy
EA 4136-Handicap et Système Nerveux, Bordeaux University; INCIA—Bordeaux University, UMR 5287 CNRS, Bordeaux, France

J. Gallinat
University Clinic Hamburg-Eppendorf, Clinic and Polyclinic for Psychiatry and Psychotherapy, Hamburg, Germany

C.A. Hanlon
Medical University of South Carolina, Charleston, SC, United States

J.Y. Hong
SRI International, Menlo Park, CA, United States

J. Jacobus
University of California, San Diego, La Jolla; VA San Diego Healthcare System, San Diego, CA, United States

J.L. Jones
Medical University of South Carolina, Charleston, SC, United States

E. Kalon
Palo Alto University, Palo Alto; SRI International, Menlo Park, CA, United States

S. Kühn
University Clinic Hamburg-Eppendorf, Clinic and Polyclinic for Psychiatry and Psychotherapy, Hamburg; Center for Lifespan Psychology, Max Planck Institute for Human Development, Berlin, Germany

M.N. Potenza
Yale University, New Haven, CT, United States

T. Schulte
Palo Alto University, Palo Alto; SRI International, Menlo Park, CA, United States

S. Tapert
University of California, San Diego, La Jolla, CA, United States

L.F. Tófoli
School of Medical Sciences, University of Campinas, Campinas, Brazil

C. Tobin
Palo Alto University, Palo Alto; National Center for PTSD, VA Palo Alto Health Care System Menlo Park Division, Menlo Park, CA, United States

PREFACE

In considering topics for this issue of the *International Review on Neurobiology*, we included work evaluating drugs of abuse, namely alcohol, stimulants (such as cocaine), and marijuana, and compulsive behaviors, notably sex, food, and gambling. Addiction to nearly all substances is diagnosed based on common criteria (Table 1), which can readily be applied to behavioral addictions.

In addition to classifying Substance Use Disorders, the Diagnostic and Statistical Manual of Mental Disorders (DSM-5) now includes gambling as an independent condition in a new category on behavioral addictions. The American Psychiatric Association chose not to include sex addiction as a distinct diagnostic category, noting that, as with "food addiction," these relatively new concepts require further investigation before inclusion as distinct diagnostic categories. Behavioral, or "chemical-free," addictions nevertheless offer a useful view of the addicted brain independent of the presence of a drug.

This volume presents diverse and unique perspectives on addiction from the viewpoint of neuroimaging.

Maud Dupuy and Sandra Chanraud review neuroimaging of Alcohol Use Disorders with an emphasis on disrupted brain connectivity and compensatory mechanisms, often mediated by the cerebellum, as reported in studies using Diffusion Tensor Imaging (DTI) and resting-state functional magnetic resonance imaging (rsfMRI).

Ty Brumback, Norma Castro, Joanna Jacobus, and Susan Tapert review neuroimaging of marijuana use with a focus on adolescence. They note that this critical neurodevelopmental period is especially vulnerable to exposure to drugs of abuse, which can significantly alter the trajectory of brain maturation.

Simone Kühn and Jürgen Gallinat review the neurobiological basis of sex addiction, maintaining that use of an unbiased term such as "hypersexuality" will help advance our understanding of the brains of individuals with persistent, socially deviant, maladaptive sexual behavior.

Ember Kalon, Jui-Yang Hong, Chelsea Tobin, and Tilman Schulte establish a theoretical framework from which to evaluate food addiction, review fMRI studies of obesity and food-cue reactivity, and highlight the relevance of the hypothalamus to brain homeostasis.

Iris Balodis and Marc Potenza review brain responses to cue and reward processing fMRI tasks to derive mechanisms of cognitive compromise in gambling disorder.

Table 1 DSM-V Criteria for Diagnosing Substance Use Disorders

1. Substance is often taken in larger amounts over a longer period of time than was intended
2. Persistent desire or unsuccessful effort to cut down or control use
3. Excessive time spent in activities necessary to obtain, use, or recover from substance
4. Craving or a strong desire to use the substance
5. Recurrent use resulting in failure to fulfill major obligations at work, school, home
6. Continued use despite having persistent or recurrent social or interpersonal problems
7. Important social, occupational, or recreational activities are given up or reduced because of substance use
8. Tolerance, as defined by either of the following:
a. A need for markedly increased amounts of the substance to achieve intoxication or desired effect
b. A markedly diminished effect with continued use of the same amount of substance
9. Withdrawal, as manifested by either of the following:
a. Characteristic withdrawal syndrome for the substance
b. Use of the substance or closely related substance is taken to relieve or avoid withdrawal symptoms

Colleen Hanlon, Logan Dowdle, and Jennifer Jones, in addition to reviewing imaging studies of the brain on cocaine, consider current studies evaluating the use of transcranial magnetic stimulation (TMS) to treat addiction.

Luís Fernando Tófoli and Draulio Barros de Araujo review electroencephalogram studies of psychedelics conducted in the early 1960s, report on the current "psychedelic renaissance," and underscore the potential of psychedelics to be used in a controlled therapeutic setting to treat addiction.

What emerges from these contributions is that neuroimaging, which permits in vivo, whole-brain analysis of the human condition, has revealed that brains of individuals with an addiction diagnosis, irrespective of substance or behavior, show alterations in overlapping brain systems, including reward, stress, and executive control networks.

The relation between drugs of abuse and the brain's reward circuitry, first explored in the 1950s, has remained a central focus of addiction research.

The term *reward system* refers to a group of structures that respond to rewarding or reinforcing stimuli. When exposed to a relevant stimulus (eg, drugs of abuse), the brain responds by increasing the release of the neurotransmitter dopamine, which is associated with the experience of a "high" or feelings of euphoria. The mesolimbic dopamine system includes dopamine-producing structures (eg, ventral tegmental area) and dopamine-responsive structures (eg, ventral striatum/nucleus accumbens). A consistent finding in the addicted brain is that continued use or exposure reduces dopamine receptor expression in areas such as the nucleus accumbens, thereby reducing the reward response to the substance or behavior, a mechanism that may underlie the expression of tolerance. As use progresses to abuse, the rewarding properties of the drug become less salient and drug taking becomes guided instead by conditioned responses (ie, habit) likely mediated by more dorsal aspects of the striatum.

A considerable body of work now supports the concept of the addicted brain as having a stress surfeit, often during withdrawal, and generally associated with dysregulation of the brain's limbic system. In the transition to addiction, motivation shifts from desire to experience the positive effects of the drug or behavior to avoidance of the negative effects, such as those that accompany withdrawal. The brain in withdrawal, associated with irritability, physical and emotional pain, dysphoria, and a loss of motivation for natural rewards, responds to stress-related chemicals such glucocorticoids, corticotropin-releasing factor (CRF), norepinephrine, and dynorphin. CRF- and dynorphin-producing neurons are present in a number of brain regions: neuroimaging research has principally focused on the amygdala, which appears to be hyperactive in the addicted brain.

The addicted brain also shows deficits in the functioning of the executive control system, governing cognitive functions including decision-making, working memory, outcome expectation, and planning. The frontally based, executive control system targets many cortical, subcortical, and diffuse neurotransmitter systems, including dopaminergic, noradrenergic, serotoninergic, and cholinergic neurons in the basal forebrain and brainstem. Engagement of frontal executive systems early in the addiction process in response to irregular activity in the brain's reward and stress systems may contribute to the transition from casual to compulsive behavior. Later in addiction, compromise of the executive system, including prefrontal, orbitofrontal, and anterior cingulate cortices, may result in loss of control, failure of self-regulation, poor decision-making, and impulsivity.

This special issue of the *International Review of Neurobiology* concludes with chapters focused on treating addiction. While still in its infancy, research examining the brain's response to TMS and psychedelic therapy holds promise for assisting individuals in overcoming addiction. An FDA-approved treatment for major depressive disorder since 2008, TMS is currently being evaluated as a treatment for a number of substance use disorders. TMS targets to reduce craving include the nucleus accumbens and prefrontal cortex. Psychedelics may be beneficial in a comprehensive treatment setting as they are serotonin receptor agonists: a number of addictive behaviors, including hypersexuality, appear to respond to selective serotonin reuptake inhibitors, which, like psychedelics, effectively increase serotonergic activity in the brain.

From our perspective as editors of this issue, other brain regions relevant to the addicted brain require additional investigation. In particular, the cerebellum, which appears to compensate for functional impairments in alcohol use disorders, has not been systemically investigated in neuroimaging studies of nonalcohol substance use disorders or in behavioral addictions. Similarly, although relevant to regulating a number of addictive-like behaviors and germane to rodent studies of addiction, the hypothalamus, likely due to its small size and location, is relatively understudied with current neuroimaging methods. Further investigation of the developing adolescent brain is also necessary as it is anticipated that such studies will help distinguish a brain at risk for from a brain already hijacked by addiction. Individual differences in vulnerability to drugs and the transition to addiction also require further scrutiny.

Finally, we would like to thank each of the authors who have contributed timely and thoughtful reviews on "Imaging the Addicted Brain." It was a pleasure to serve as editors for this volume of the *International Review of Neurobiology* and we predict that researchers and clinicians alike will find this resource a comprehensive guide to a biologically based understanding of the addicted brain.

Conflict of interest: The authors declare no competing financial interest in relation to the work described here.

Natalie M. Zahr
Neuroscience Program,
SRI International,
Menlo Park, CA, United States

Psychiatry & Behavioral Sciences,
Stanford University School of Medicine,
Stanford, CA, United States

Eric T. Peterson
Neuroscience Program,
SRI International,
Menlo Park, CA, United States

CHAPTER ONE

Imaging the Addicted Brain: Alcohol

M. Dupuy[*,†,1], **S. Chanraud**[‡]
[*]EA 4136-Handicap et Système Nerveux, Bordeaux University, Bordeaux, France
[†]INCIA—Bordeaux University, UMR 5287 CNRS, Bordeaux, France
[‡]EPHE, PSL Research University, Bordeaux, France
[1]Corresponding author: e-mail address: maud.dupuy@u-bordeaux.fr

Contents

Abstract

Alcohol use disorder (AUD) represents a major public health issue due to its prevalence and severe health consequences. It may affect several aspects of an individual's life including work and relationships, and it also increases risk for additional problems such as brain injury. The causes and outcomes of AUD are varied; thus, attempting to understand this complex phenomenon requires investigation from multiple perspectives. Magnetic resonance imaging (MRI) is a powerful means to investigate brain anatomical and functional alterations related to AUD. Recent advances in MRI methods allow better investigation of the alterations to structural and functional brain networks in AUD. Here, we focus on findings from studies using multiple MRI techniques, which converge to support the considerable vulnerability of frontal systems. Indeed, MRI studies provide evidence for a "disconnection syndrome" which could be involved in the poor behavioral control observed in AUD.

International Review of Neurobiology, Volume 129
ISSN 0074-7742
http://dx.doi.org/10.1016/bs.irn.2016.04.003

1. ALCOHOL USE DISORDER: DEFINITION, EPIDEMIOLOGY, AND CONSEQUENCES

1.1 Definitions

Alcohol is a psychoactive substance with dependence-producing properties. In most cultures, it is the most frequently used intoxicating substance. The definition of alcohol use disorder (AUD) has varied over the years. In the fourth edition of the *Diagnostic and Statistical Manual of Mental Disorders* (4th ed., text revision; DSM-IV-TR; American Psychiatric Association, 2000), the diagnoses included categories of "alcohol abuse" and "alcohol dependence," each with specific criteria. The fifth edition, DSM-5 (5th ed., DSM-5; American Psychiatric Association, 2013), combines the two DSM-IV categories of "alcohol abuse" and "alcohol dependence" into one disorder called AUD, measured on a continuum from mild to severe, according to number of criteria met. In the DSM-5, recurrent legal problems as a criterion for alcohol abuse was removed, as it was a difficult criterion to apply internationally, considering differences in legal practices; a new criterion—craving or a strong desire to use alcohol—was added. It was noted that the diagnostic term of "dependence" is confusing. Indeed, "dependence" and "addiction" are two terms that are often used interchangeably, even though they refer to different phenomena. According to the American Psychiatric Association (2013) "dependence can be a normal body response to a substance." The term "addiction" is not considered in the Diagnostic and Statistical Manuals of Mental Disorders as it has an uncertain definition and is potentially associated with a negative connotation.

Regardless of the exact definition used, substance-related disorders are complex phenomena that have various interpretations in the literature. They have an array of causes and consequences that may cooccur with other chronic diseases and affect various facets of an individual's life, family, and community, as well as society as a whole. The understanding of these phenomena constitutes a broad field of study that spans several disciplines and approaches. The scientific findings reported in this chapter mainly deal with alcohol dependence, as defined by DSM-IV-TR, and with AUD, as it is described in the DSM-5, and additionally relate results concerning abstinence and relapse.

1.2 Epidemiology

Estimating the prevalence of AUD is difficult considering differences in research methodology and changes in the diagnostic criteria over the years. In 2010 however, the worldwide prevalence of AUD among individuals aged 15 years and older was estimated at 4%, with the highest prevalence rates found in Europe (in line with the International Statistical Classification of Diseases and Related Health Problem 10th Revision's definition of dependence and harmful use of alcohol; ICD-10; WHO, 2014). AUD appears, therefore, to be a very common disorder, significantly more prevalent among men, but affecting people of all ages and socioeconomic groups.

1.3 Consequences

The evolution of AUD is variable and can include periods of remission and relapse. AUD may impair several major aspects of individual's life functioning. It is associated with health risks, including fetal damage when pregnant mothers drink, hypertension, liver and heart disease, depression, neurological deficits, and can be fatal. The harmful use of alcohol is one of the world's leading health risks, resulting in approximately 2.5 million preventable deaths each year (WHO, 2010). In addition, AUD may also affect behavioral, occupational, social, and economic dimensions of an individual's daily life. It is associated with a significant increase in the risk of injuries, accidents (car- and job-related accidents), violence, and suicide (Singh et al., 2015; WHO, 2011). AUD may also impact individuals' family members. This can result in, but is not limited to, having unmet developmental needs, impaired attachment, economic hardship, legal problems, emotional distress, and violence (Lander, Howsare, & Byrne, 2013). AUD has a strong comorbidity with other psychiatric conditions especially bipolar disorders, schizophrenia, and antisocial personality disorder; but also, anxiety, and depressive disorders (Marshall & Farrell, 2007).

On a societal level, AUD can also be costly to communities. Economically, this manifests in prevention and treatment costs, health care and hospital costs, increased morbidity, and mortality. In the majority of countries worldwide (53.9%), alcohol was identified as the main substance of abuse at entry into treatment (WHO, 2010). This disorder is also of concern to victims of alcohol-related violence and accidents. Finally, an additional cost of AUD to take into account is the decrease of employee productivity (Bouchery, Harwood, Sacks, Simon, & Brewer, 2011).

1.4 Imaging the Brain

There are several powerful methods to image both the structure and function of the brain, and many have been used to gain a better understanding the neurobiological underpinnings of AUD. Among them, morphometric magnetic resonance imaging (MRI) provides a noninvasive means of exploring of the shape, size, and integrity of gray and white matter (WM) macrostructure of the brain. Diffusion tensor imaging (DTI) is commonly used to assess WM microstructure of the brain. DTI allows for the exploration of structural connectivity between different brain regions by measuring the spatially preferential diffusion of water molecules in WM tracts of the brain. Functional magnetic resonance imaging (fMRI) allows for the exploration of brain activity by taking advantage of local metabolism. fMRI detects "activation" of specific brain regions, while an individual is performing a task (eg, cognitive or sensorimotor) related to a local increase in oxygen consumption, based on changes in regional deoxyhemoglobin concentrations in the brain. This fMRI signal is called the blood-oxygen-level-dependent (BOLD) effect, and its changes are used to determine which brain regions are involved in a particular task (Norris, 2006). fMRI is also capable of mapping functionally related brain networks by measuring correlated activity of different regions, ie, functional connectivity (FC). A constellation of brain regions may have highly correlated spontaneous activity even when a subject is not engaged in a specific task (Biswal, Yetkin, Haughton, & Hyde, 1995), and much of the brain's energy is consumed by spontaneous activity (Fox & Raichle, 2007). These observations were the impetus for pursuing so-called resting-state fMRI, conducted at rest, without task demands, and using complex correlational approaches to explore the intrinsic FC of the brain (Beckmann, DeLuca, Devlin, & Smith, 2005). It is now evident that brain regions are organized into intrinsic networks (Allen et al., 2011) with the most representative resting-state network referred to as the "default mode network" (DMN), a network that is activated at rest, but turns off (is deactivated) while performing a task (Ferreira & Busatto, 2013; Raichle et al., 2001). Regions considered part of the DMN include the posterior cingulate cortex, retrosplenial cortex, inferior parietal cortex, medial prefrontal cortex, the medial temporal lobe (Buckner, Andrews-Hanna, & Schacter, 2008a, 2008b), and the precuneus (Margulies et al., 2009). This chapter will focus on results from studies using the above-mentioned MRI tools, but is by no means exhaustive. Results of other imaging modalities (eg, magnetic resonance spectroscopy and positron emission tomography) are not discussed here.

2. STRUCTURAL BRAIN IMAGING IN AUD

2.1 Macrostructural Brain Imaging in AUD

CT scans provided the "first" evidence of AUD-related brain alterations, followed quickly by structural MRI scans. Several analyses methods are available for investigating the morphology of the brain from data acquired using MRI. A widely used analysis tool is voxel-based morphometry (VBM; Ashburner & Friston, 2000). In VBM, all images from all the subjects in the study are spatially normalized into the same stereotactic space. Individuals' structural brain images are then segmented into gray matter (GM), WM, and cerebrospinal fluid and finally smoothed. Voxelwise parametric statistical tests are performed on gray matter images from the two groups to compare brain regional volumes. The output of VBM is a statistical parametric map revealing between group differences in brain regional volumes or densities of gray matter.

VBM has been used to investigate morphological differences between brains of individuals with AUD and healthy controls (Chanraud et al., 2007; Mechtcheriakov et al., 2007; Rando et al., 2011). One of the first studies explored GM and WM volume in 22 alcohol-dependent patients compared to 22 healthy controls matched for age and sex. In patients with alcohol dependence, a decrease in GM volume was found in frontal cortical areas, posterior hippocampus, and thalamus. VBM conducted on WM revealed reduced volume in a periventricular area, the pons, and cerebellum (Fig. 1).

A more recent study compared GM volume in 45, 1-month abstinent, alcohol-dependent patients, and 50 healthy volunteers. In line with previous results, significant GM volume loss in alcohol-dependent patients relative to comparison subjects was found in the lateral prefrontal cortex, the medial frontal cortex, and the posterior cingulate gyrus.

Similar findings are widely reported, regardless of the methods used for analysis. Alterations of GM seem particularly localized in focal regions such as the frontal cortex, the thalamus, the insular cortex, the dorsal hippocampus, and the cerebellum (Cardenas, Studholme, Gazdzinski, Durazzo, & Meyerhoff, 2007; Grodin, Lin, Durkee, Hommer, & Momenan, 2013), while alterations in WM are widespread and include the corpus callosum, frontotemporal regions, periventricular areas, pons, and cerebellum (Chanraud et al., 2007). Fortier et al. (2011) used a very sensitive and accurate whole-brain cortical thickness analysis, not limited by arbitrary anatomical boundaries (without a priori definitions of regions of interest [ROI]). This approach has advantages in detecting regionally specific cortical atrophy across the full cortical surface without being limited by traditional a priori regional hypotheses. The authors demonstrated that individuals with AUD have decreased whole-brain cortical thickness as compared to nonalcoholic control participants.

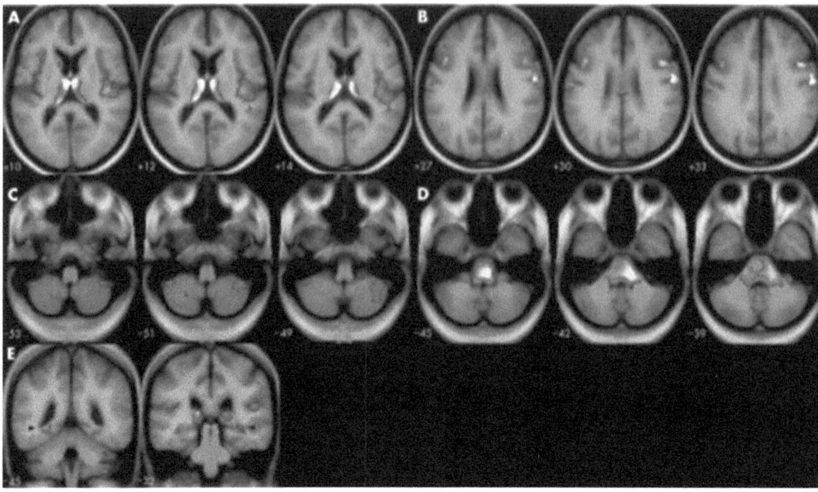

Fig. 1 Areas of significant gray and white matter decrease in patients with alcohol addiction relative to healthy controls. Results are illustrated as statistical parametric map blobs superimposed on the slices of a T1-weighted mean picture in standard stereotactic space from all 44 study participants. The *left side* of the figure is the *left side* of the brain. Threshold was set at $p > 3.31$ (peak). (A) Thalamus, insula; (B) middle frontal gyrus, precentral gyrus; (C) cerebellum; (D) brainstem; and (E) dorsal hippocampus. *From Mechtcheriakov, S., Brenneis, C., Egger, K., Koppelstaetter, F., Schocke, M., & Marksteiner, J. (2007). A widespread distinct pattern of cerebral atrophy in patients with alcohol addiction revealed by voxel-based morphometry.* Journal of Neurology, Neurosurgery and Psychiatry, *78(6), 610.*

Thus, AUD has been associated with extensive GM and WM damage. The specific regions affected by AUD are presented later (Cardenas et al., 2007; Grodin et al., 2013; Harper & Matsumoto, 2005; Mechtcheriakov et al., 2007; Moselhy, Georgiou, & Kahn, 2001; Pfefferbaum, Desmond, et al., 2001; Pfefferbaum, Rosenbloom, Deshmukh, & Sullivan, 2001). Morphometric analysis has revealed smaller volumes of regions in brain reward networks in AUD subjects (Makris et al., 2008). Volume deficits were found in right dorsolateral prefrontal cortex, right anterior insula, right nucleus accumbens, and left amygdala. Such damage in the brain reward system could precede the onset of alcoholism, be the result of chronic drinking, or represent an interaction.

2.1.1 Corpus Callosum

Decreased volume of the corpus callosum in alcoholic subjects relative to controls was demonstrated several times, with thinning being more prominent in anterior than posterior regions (Estruch et al., 1997; Pfefferbaum, Lim, Desmond, & Sullivan, 1996; Ruiz et al., 2013). There is also evidence for gender-related effects of alcoholism on corpus callosum volumes. It appears that alcoholic men are more sensitive to corpus callosum damage, whereas frontal and temporal WM areas are more sensitive in alcoholic women (Ruiz et al., 2013).

2.1.2 Insula

Shape analysis (Jung et al., 2007; Makris et al., 2008) and volumetric (Chanraud et al., 2007) methods have revealed differences in the insula of alcoholics compared with controls. Shape deformations were mainly localized in the central part of the insula in both hemispheres, with a greater difference in the right than in the left hemisphere. In healthy subjects, the surface of left insula is more convex than the right one, suggesting that the left–right insula asymmetry observed in healthy subjects is reduced in alcoholics (Jung et al., 2007).

2.1.3 Striatum

Some MRI studies have revealed smaller volumes of caudate and putamen in alcoholics than in controls, regardless of length of sobriety (Boutte, 2012; Sullivan, Deshmukh, De Rosa, Rosenbloom, & Pfefferbaum, 2005). In a more recent study, the nucleus accumbens was shown to have greater volume shrinkage in more recent than longer sober alcoholics (Sullivan et al., 2005).

2.1.4 Hippocampus

Structural neuroimaging studies have demonstrated hippocampal volume deficits in alcoholics (Agartz, Momenan, Rawlings, Kerich, & Hommer, 1999; Kurth et al., 2004; Laakso et al., 2000; Sullivan, Marsh, Mathalon, Lim, & Pfefferbaum, 1995; Wilhelm et al., 2008). Hippocampal volume shrinkage has been attributed to pathological changes in WM (eg, decrease in axonal diameter; Harding, Wong, Svoboda, Kril, & Halliday, 1997), but the incorporation of newly formed neurons to the dentate gyrus also appears to be affected by alcohol (He et al., 2005; Nixon & Crews, 2004). Comparing late-onset alcoholics (Type I), violent, early-onset alcoholics (Type II), and non-alcoholic controls (Laakso et al., 2000), the right but not the left hippocampus was significantly smaller in both alcoholic groups. Despite the absence of age-related decline in hippocampal volumes in the control subjects (Sullivan et al., 2005), alcoholics with Type I showed a tendency toward decreased volumes with age, and also with the duration of alcoholism (Laakso et al., 2000). In another study comparing alcoholics with nonalcoholic controls, left hippocampal volume reduction was slightly greater than on the right (Beresford et al., 2006). The type of alcoholic beverage consumed appears to have an effect on hippocampal volume, with a stronger negative correlation found in subjects consuming wine and spirits than in subjects consuming beer, indicating that more concentrated alcohol reduces hippocampal volume more significantly (Wilhelm et al., 2008). The effects of different types of alcoholic beverages on hippocampus may be accounted for by homocysteine-mediated excitotoxicity. Indeed, homocysteine is a mediator of excitotoxicity and neurotoxicity via overstimulation of NMDA receptors (Lipton et al., 1997) and its plasma concentration is dependent on both the type of beverage and amount of alcohol consumed (Bleich et al., 2003).

2.1.5 Amygdala

Using a modified version of VBM analysis, Fein et al. (2006) specifically examined the amygdala in abstinent alcoholics who demonstrated impairment on a simulated gambling task. It has been demonstrated that amygdala and ventromedial prefrontal regions are required for optimal performance on this task. Compared with controls, abstinent alcoholics had significantly less GM in the amygdala. The authors were cautious in attributing this dysmorphology to alcoholism per se and offered an alternative explanation that the structural abnormality predated alcoholism. Given the amygdala's role in emotional regulation and behavioral control (for review, see McBride, 2002), premorbid deficits in these functions (due to smaller volumes) could put individuals at heightened risk for developing AUD (Clark, Thatcher, & Tapert, 2008; Kamarajan et al., 2006). In addition to being smaller, amygdala volume was negatively associated with both alcohol craving and probability of relapse within 6 months following detoxification (Wrase et al., 2008).

2.1.6 Brainstem

Brain regions that are part of the brainstem have been observed by MRI and found to be altered in alcoholic men (Bloomer, Langleben, & Meyerhoff, 2004; Sullivan & Marsh, 2003) and women (Pfefferbaum, Rosenbloom, Serventi, & Sullivan, 2002). More recently, these findings were confirmed for the pons with a regional investigation, whereas midbrain volume did not differ between alcoholics and controls, the volume of the pons was smaller in alcoholics than controls (Chanraud et al., 2007).

2.1.7 Cerebellum

The cerebellum, like the frontal lobes, is one of the primary brain targets of alcohol's devastating effects (Harper, 1998). Subjects with AUD show smaller cerebellar GM volume (Boutte et al., 2012). MRI studies have also revealed in the cerebellar vermis a 33% volume deficit in chronic alcoholics (Antunez et al., 1998); damages appeared predominantly in anterior superior but not posterior inferior regions (Sullivan, Deshmukh, Desmond, Lim, & Pfefferbaum, 2000). This is of particular interest given recent data showing the importance of the cerebellum in the organization of higher order cerebral functions and its structural connections with the frontal lobe (Balsters & Ramnani, 2011; Balsters, Whelan, Robertson, & Ramnani, 2013; Sullivan & Marsh, 2003).

2.2 Microstructural Brain Imaging in AUD

WM abnormalities are considered a characteristic of AUD, with atrophy reported in postmortem and neuroimaging studies (Zahr, 2014). DTI, which allows in vivo quantitative characterization of WM microstructure, and thus brain *structural* connectivity, has also revealed microstructural impairment related to AUD. Fractional anisotropy (FA) is a DTI metric used to describe axonal integrity and myelination. It represents the proportion of nonrandom (ie, anisotropic) diffusion of water molecules in a voxel. It ranges between 0, isotropic diffusion, and 1, total anisotropic diffusion. More specifically, it is an index of fiber diameter and density, degree of myelination, extracellular diffusion, interaxonal spacing, and intravoxel fiber-tract coherence. Higher FA may reflect effective myelination and integrity of fibers (coherence of fiber orientation, increased axonal density, and decreased axonal diameter) (Jones, Knösche, & Turner, 2013).

There is consistency in the literature regarding alteration of five fibers tracts in AUDs: body of corpus callosum, fornix, external capsule, cingulate gyrus, and superior longitudinal fasciculus (Fig. 2; Monnig et al., 2015; Pfefferbaum, Adalsteinsson, & Sullivan, 2006; Pfefferbaum, Rosenbloom, Rohlfing, & Sullivan, 2009; Yeh, Simpson, Durazzo, Gazdzinski, & Meyerhoff, 2009). These WM pathways are involved in a large number of higher order functions, including visuospatial and language processing (superior longitudinal fasciculus), interhemispheric communication (corpus callosum), memory and emotional processing (fornix), decision making (cingulum), and sensory integration (external capsule).

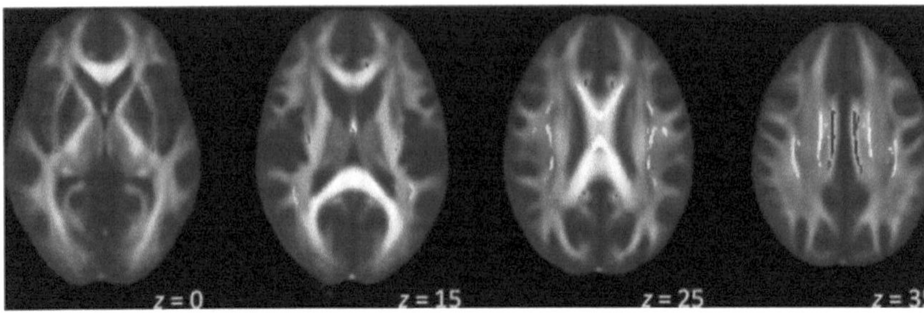

Fig. 2 Tracts included in the white matter factor (WMF), shown on FSL's FMRIB58 FA image. *Color legend*: external capsule, *red* (*gray* in the print version); fornix, *light blue* (*white* in the print version); body of corpus callosum, *yellow* (*white* in the print version); cingulate gyrus, *dark blue* (*dark gray* in the print version); and superior longitudinal fasciculus, *green* (*light gray* in the print version). *From Monnig, M. A., Yeo, R. A., Tonigan, J. S., McCrady, B. S., Thoma, R. J., Sabbineni, A., & Hutchison, K. E. (2015). Associations of white matter microstructure with clinical and demographic characteristics in heavy drinkers.* PloS One, 10*(11), e0142042. http://doi.org/10.1371/journal.pone.0142042.*

Studies have shown widespread FA deficits in both hemispheres of alcoholic subjects (Pfefferbaum et al., 2006) as well as WM tract damage in the genu and splenium of the corpus callosum, the centrum semiovale (Pfefferbaum, Adalsteinsson, & Sullivan, 2005; Pfefferbaum et al., 2002; Pfefferbaum et al., 2000), corticopontine bundles (Chanraud et al., 2009), and right frontolimbic connections (Harris et al., 2008). Alcohol-dependent subjects have lower FA in the fornix, anterior commissure, and right inferior frontooccipital fasciculus, regions implicated in emotional processing, cognition, and executive functioning (Durkee, Sarlls, Hommer, & Momenan, 2013).

Although WM changes related to AUD are well established, identifying vulnerability factors such as disorder severity, drinking behavior, or demographic characteristics requires further investigation. Some studies have reported greater alcohol-related WM damage in women (Mann, Schäfer, Längle, Ackermann, & Croissant, 2005), older (Pfefferbaum et al., 2006), and treatment-seeking (Gazdzinski, Durazzo, Weiner, & Meyerhoff, 2008) individuals, but other studies have not reported such relationships (Pfefferbaum, Desmond, et al., 2001; Pfefferbaum, Rosenbloom, et al., 2001). Monnig et al. (2015) investigated the impact of chronic alcohol exposure on WM microstructure as a function of AUD severity, recent drinking behavior, and demographic characteristics. They showed that AUD severity and drinking frequency were significant predictors of lower WM FA in the corpus callosum, external capsule, cingulate gyrus, superior longitudinal fasciculus, and fornix. Consistent with previous studies (eg, Mann et al., 2005; Pfefferbaum et al., 2009), they demonstrated that women have lower FA in these five tracts of interest and that more frequent drinking contributed to lower FA in women but not men, suggesting a gender-specific vulnerability to alcohol's WM toxicity. They also observed a main effect of age on FA in which the older group had overall lower FA values.

Alterations in DTI measures of WM may underlie cognitive and emotional deficits observed in AUD (Durkee et al., 2013). WM impairments could lead to altered communication between GM regions which function together as brain networks. Alcohol-dependent subjects exhibit difficulties in decision making, particularly in decisions related to emotional and motivated behaviors. DTI studies have detected WM impairments in neural systems associated with reward seeking, emotional processing, and cognitive control (Monnig et al., 2013; Yeh et al., 2009). In alcohol-dependent subjects, correlated with alterations in WM are impairments in visuospatial abilities (Müller-Oehring, Schulte, Fama, Pfefferbaum, & Sullivan, 2009), cognitive flexibility (Chanraud et al., 2009), executive functions (Chanraud et al., 2007), balance, and psychomotor speed (Pfefferbaum, Rosenbloom, Fama, Sassoon, & Sullivan, 2010). These weakened or abnormal connections provide evidence for a "disconnection syndrome" in AUD (Geschwind, 2010).

3. FUNCTIONAL BRAIN IMAGING IN AUD

3.1 Activation

Task-based fMRI studies have revealed that, for the same level of performance, alcoholic individuals show less activation (Chanraud, Pitel, Müller-Oehring, Pfefferbaum, & Sullivan, 2013; Desmond et al., 2003) or activate different brain regions (Pfefferbaum, Desmond, et al., 2001; Pfefferbaum, Rosenbloom, et al., 2001; Tapert et al., 2001) than control subjects. Using a spatial working memory task for which two groups of men, with and without alcoholism, perform at equivalent levels, Pfefferbaum, Desmond, et al. (2001) and Pfefferbaum, Rosenbloom, et al. (2001) demonstrated that alcoholics showed diminished activation of executive control (EC) regions (bilateral dorsolateral prefrontal cortex) compared to controls. Further, different patterns of activation were observed between groups. The control group showed appropriate activation of the dorsal (Where?) stream, involving the occipital–parietal system, known to be involved in visuospatial working memory processing. To successfully perform the spatial working memory task, the alcoholic group exhibited activation of the ventral (What?) stream, involving the inferior occipital–temporal and the limbic systems, related to declarative memory processing. Considering equivalent group performance, the authors suggested that the atypical pattern of brain activations displayed by the alcoholic group was consistent with a functional reorganization of brain systems leading to the use of alternative neural pathways to execute the task, when the usual ones are compromised. Similar results were observed in women with a history of alcoholism (Tapert et al., 2001).

Desmond et al. (2003) examined brain activation differences between alcoholic and nonalcoholic men performing a verbal working memory task. Again, despite comparable performance, analysis of the functional data revealed that the alcoholics compared to the matched controls exhibited greater activation in the left frontal (BA44/45) and right superior cerebellar (HVI) regions, regions that support the articulatory control system of verbal working memory in young healthy controls. Greater activations in alcoholics in the frontal/superior cerebellar circuit may suggest that this circuit is functionally compromised and requires a compensatory increase in activation to reach the same level of performance as controls. These results highlight the potential role of cerebellum to compensate for functional impairments in frontal regions, consistent with anatomical connections between frontal and cerebellar regions (Schmahmann & Pandya, 1997; Zahr, Pitel, Chanraud, & Sullivan, 2010).

Another study investigating the compensation hypothesis according to operationally defined criteria (Davis, Dennis, Daselaar, Fleck, & Cabeza, 2008) used a spatial working memory task (Chanraud et al., 2013). A relationship was identified between a brain region which was more activated in alcoholics than controls (dorsolateral prefrontal cortex), and a region which was less activated in recovering alcoholics than controls (cerebellar regions VI/Crus I) (Fig. 3). Despite different levels of activation, activity within cerebellar region VI was positively correlated to accuracy in both groups. This finding indicates that involvement of this region is essential for performing the task.

BOLD activity during motor performance has also been investigated in AUD. Detoxified alcohol-dependent patients and matched controls show different patterns of brain activation while performing on par on easy motor tasks (ie, externally paced (EP) and self-paced (SP) finger tapping) (Parks et al., 2010). During EP tapping, alcoholics showed a significant increase of activation in right precentral gyrus and left postcentral and temporal gyrus as compared to controls. Further, areas activated only by alcoholics included

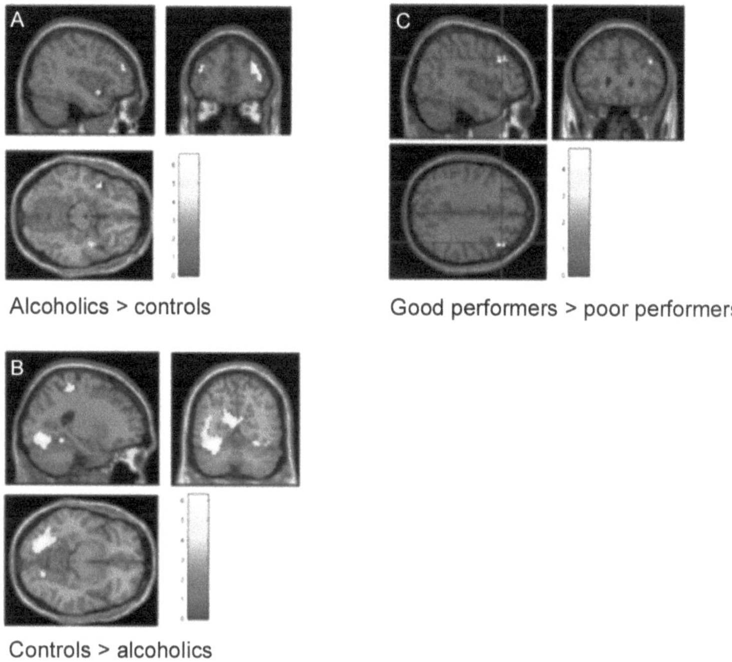

Fig. 3 *Left*: Brain regional activation in (A) alcoholics relative to controls at the *top* and (B) controls relative to alcoholics at the *bottom*, while performing on the task. (C) Brain regional activation in good alcoholics performers (eight subjects) relative to poor alcoholics performers (seven subjects). Cutoff for performance estimated with accuracy = 50% of good responses; $p < 0.05$ FDR corrected and $k > 10$ voxels. *From Chanraud, S., Pitel, A.-L., Müller-Oehring, E. M., Pfefferbaum, A., & Sullivan, E. V. (2013). Remapping the brain to compensate for impairment in recovering alcoholics.* Cerebral Cortex (New York, N.Y.: 1991), *23(1), 97–104. http://doi.org/10.1093/cercor/bhr381.*

the right postcentral and frontal gyrus and the left fusiform gyrus. However, during SP tapping, the right parietal lobule was activated significantly more in alcoholics than in controls, and the right postcentral gyrus was activated exclusively in patients. All these results indicate that patients had to recruit more brain regions to reach the same level of performance as control subjects. The authors also explored within-group differences in brain activations when contrasting EP vs SP finger tapping. During SP tapping alcoholics seemed to employ higher order (less "automatic") functions by recruiting parietal regions, which were not engaged by controls. Instead, the latter recruited corticocerebellar regions (Fig. 4) (Parks et al., 2010). These findings are consistent with impaired frontocerebellar pathways in AUD.

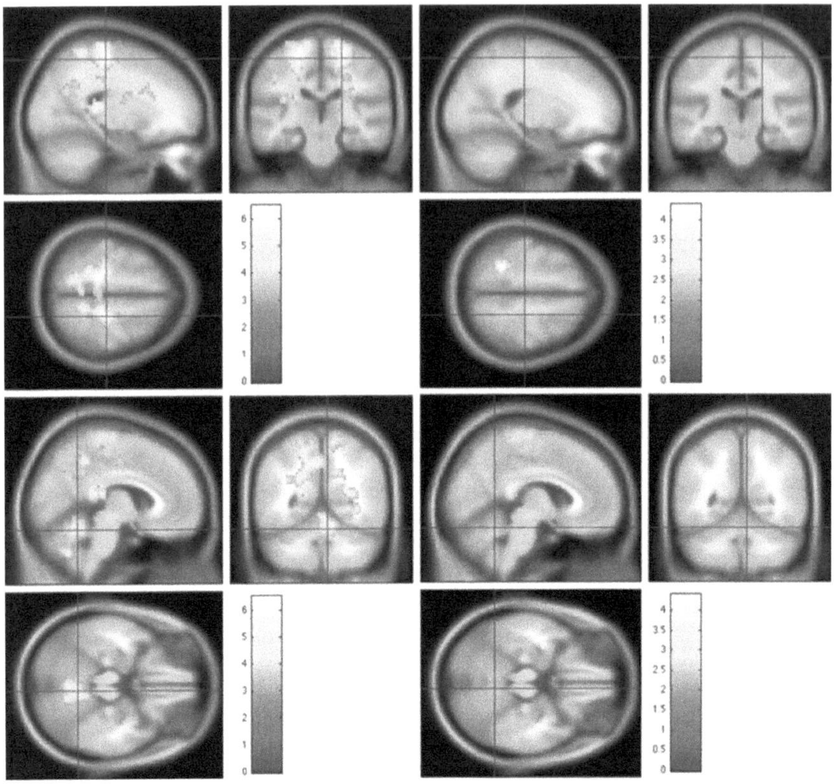

Fig. 4 Frontocerebellar activation maps in normal controls (NC, *left*) and chronic alcoholics (ALC, *right*). Differences in brain activation between self-paced (SP) and externally paced (EP) tapping performance were compared: (SP [DH & NDH combined] > EP [DH & NDH combined]). The cursor is centered on the activated voxel with the highest *Z*-score in NC for both regional representations. *Top panels*: Right BA 4 in the posterior frontal lobe (Talairach *x*18/*y* − 29/*z* − 53) in NC. The only visible activation in ALC (*right top panel*, axial view) represents the left BA 7 parietal precuneus (Talairach *x* − 24/*y* − 51/*z*50). *Bottom panels*: Right anterior cerebellar lobe (Talairach *x*5/*y* − 50/*z* − 19) in NC only. The scale of the *color* (*different gray shades* in the print version) *bars* in each panel corresponds to the statistical significance of the activation. For viewing purposes, a voxelwise threshold of $p < 0.001$ was applied. *From Parks, M. H., Greenberg, D. S., Nickel, M. K., Dietrich, M. S., Rogers, B. P., & Martin, P. R. (2010). Recruitment of additional brain regions to accomplish simple motor tasks in chronic alcohol-dependent patients.* Alcoholism, Clinical and Experimental Research, *34(6), 1098–1109. http://doi.org/10.1111/j.1530-0277.2010.01186.x.*

Neuroimaging studies have also provided evidence for compensatory mechanisms during emotional processing by chronic alcoholics (Gilman, Davis, & Hommer, 2010; Marinkovic et al., 2009). BOLD activity was investigated when subjects saw emotionally charged words and photographs of faces during deep (semantic) and shallow (perceptual) encoding tasks followed by a recognition task. Subjects were asked to perform four different encoding tasks, which varied in both type of material (faces or words) and depth of encoding (deep or shallow). Alcoholics were slower than controls in rating the emotion expressed on a face and in rating the words as abstract or concrete, but the groups did not differ in accuracy or reaction time (RT) during the recognition-testing phase. Whereas the emotional network appears to have lower responsivity to emotional cues in chronic alcoholics, it has been suggested that they may recruit prefrontal rather than temporal limbic areas when presented with emotionally or socially challenging situations (Marinkovic et al., 2009). Another study reported that alcoholics activated more frontal, limbic, and temporal regions relative to controls when they had to make judgments about whether they liked or disliked an image. Activations were higher in individuals with AUD in the frontal lobe and in areas of the brain associated with language (Gilman et al., 2010).

3.2 Functional Connectivity

In recent years, a growing interest in resting-state FC has emerged from the observation that a specific set of brain areas decrease their activity during goal-directed tasks when compared to a passive control condition such as visual fixation or eyes-closed resting (Raichle & Snyder, 2007). The presence of task-specific deactivations implied the existence of a default mode of brain function. Intrinsic, or ongoing, activity is at least as important as evoked activity by momentary environmental demands. Indeed, the cost, in terms of brain energy budget, of intrinsic activity exceeds the cost of evoked activity (for a review, see Raichle & Mintun, 2006). In addition, intrinsic activity has a significant degree of functional organization. Brain regions exhibiting spontaneous synchronized activity constitute intrinsic networks characterized by a complex activation–deactivation mechanism operating between resting state and task conditions. The DMN is considered a representative network of the rest condition. Regions in this network show a decrease in their activity during specific tasks when compared to passive resting conditions (Raichle et al., 2001; Shulman et al., 1997). The DMN includes the posterior cingulate cortex, retrosplenial cortex, inferior parietal cortex, medial prefrontal cortex, the medial temporal lobe (Buckner et al., 2008a, 2008b), and the precuneus (Margulies et al., 2009). It is now assumed that all brain areas have a high level of organized default functional activity. Alterations of one or several of these intrinsic networks as a consequence of AUD may interfere with behavior (Andrews-Hanna et al., 2007; Chanraud, Pitel, Pfefferbaum, & Sullivan, 2011).

The DMN was the first intrinsic functional network reported as disrupted in chronic alcoholism (Chanraud et al., 2011). At rest, the spontaneous fluctuations of fMRI signals in the left posterior cingulate and cerebellar regions in short-term abstinent alcoholics were less synchronized than in controls, revealing compromised FC. DMN brain areas are normally highly correlated during rest and intra-DMN connectivity is supposed to decrease during performance of a task (Buckner et al., 2008a, 2008b; Marrelec & Fransson, 2011). This functional decoupling is probably necessary for efficient processing by enabling allocation of brain resources to appropriate regions. This abnormal synchrony was interpreted as potentially reflecting processing inefficiency and disrupted connectivity precluding direct transmission between brain regions consistent with pathophysiological models of alcoholism providing new evidence for a "disconnection syndrome" in AUD (Chanraud et al., 2011; Chanraud, Zahr, Sullivan, & Pfefferbaum, 2010; Geschwind, 2010). Moreover, in the same study, it was observed that during a spatial working memory task, on which alcoholics performed equally with controls, connectivity between the left posterior cingulate seed and left cerebellar regions (IV/V) was greater in alcohol-dependent subjects than in controls (Fig. 5). The cerebellar Lobule IV/V is a region outside of the DMN, usually involved in motor functions.

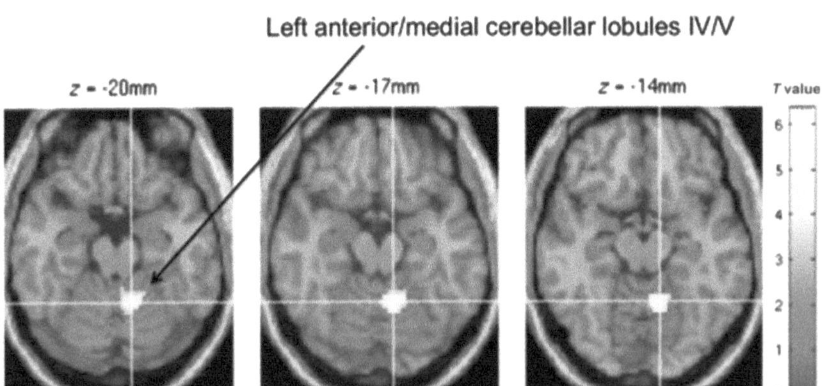

Fig. 5 Between-group comparison of the functional connectivity during the task with the left posterior cingulate cortex as seed. $p < 0.05$ FDR corrected. *From Chanraud, S., Pitel, A.-L., Pfefferbaum, A., & Sullivan, E. V. (2011). Disruption of functional connectivity of the default-mode network in alcoholism.* Cerebral Cortex (New York, N.Y.: 1991), *21(10), 2272–2281. http://doi.org/10.1093/cercor/bhq297.*

The presence of extrafunctional connections outside the DMN together with the observation of comparable performance between groups led the authors to hypothesize that a compensatory mechanism could operate through an alternative network, to compensate for a compromised network.

The cerebellum seems to be particularly involved in AUD, either as a vulnerable brain region or as a region engaged in compensation phenomena. On the other hand, evidence from a number of studies suggests that dysfunction of cortico-thalamo-cerebellar circuitry may be a major predisposing factor for alcoholism (Tessner & Hill, 2010). Since finger movements require frontal and cerebellar systems, finger tapping is a simple and easily implemented task permitting exploration of the integrity of frontocerebellar circuits. By focusing on regions that exhibited an fMRI response associated with this task in alcoholic patients, Rogers, Parks, Nickel, Katwal, and Martin (2012) showed reduced frontocerebellar FC in recently abstinent alcoholic patients compared to healthy controls. Connectivity in alcoholics was reduced between prefrontal cortex (Brodmann Area 9) and Lobule VIII of inferior cerebellum, and between premotor areas (Brodmann Area 6) and Lobule VI of superior cerebellum (Fig. 6). Such results support the hypothesis that dysfunction of the frontocerebellar circuit is particularly relevant in alcoholism.

During a task engaging executive functions (ie, Stroop task), Schulte, Müller-Oehring, Sullivan, and Pfefferbaum (2012) observed that connectivity of the middle cingulate cortex (MCC) was modified in alcoholics compared to controls. For this experiment, the Stroop effect was defined as the difference in RT between incongruent and congruent stimuli. The results suggest that alcoholics did not benefit from response repetitions and valid color cueing in congruent trials. FC in regions showing significant group-by-task activation contrast was investigated, and the analysis revealed that whereas MCC connectivity with the posterior cingulate (striatal) and medial prefrontal cortices was attenuated in alcoholics, the MCC connectivity with the midbrain and orbitofrontal regions was heightened. Enhanced midbrain–MCC connectivity in alcoholics, particularly for more difficult task conditions, implied that functional recovery may be mediated through network adaptation or reorganization. The authors interpreted these findings as reflecting neurofunctional compensation, similar to recruitment of additional brain regions, beyond those normally needed to accomplish the task. Low inhibitory control and high impulsivity seem to be implicated in the development and maintenance of alcohol dependence. In an alcohol-dependent sample exclusively, Courtney, Ghahremani, and Ray (2013)

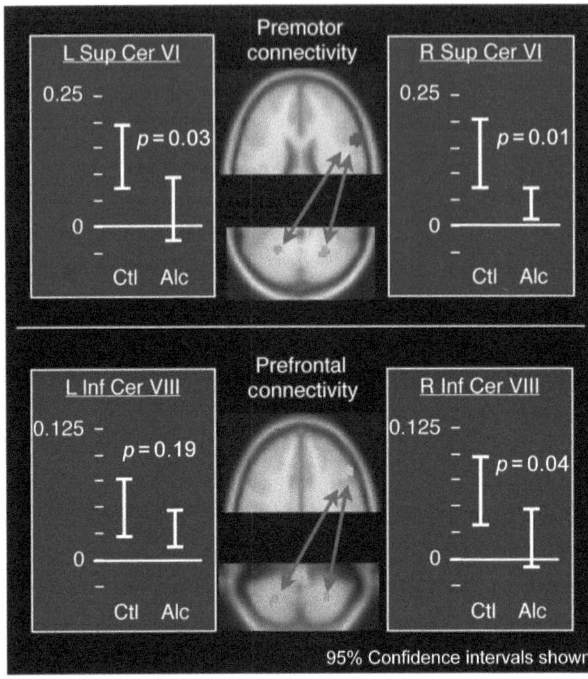

Fig. 6 Frontocerebellar functional connectivity was lower in alcoholic patients than in matched healthy controls. The seed regions are indicated in *blue* (*dark gray* in the print version) (premotor) and *green* (*light gray* in the print version) (prefrontal); the cerebellar target regions are *magenta* (*gray* in the print version). The alcoholic patients exhibited a significant reduction in connectivity between premotor cortex and Lobule VI in superior cerebellum, and between prefrontal cortex and Lobule VIII in inferior cerebellum. Connectivity between a number of other regions did not differ between patients and controls, suggesting that the result was specific to frontocerebellar circuits. *From Rogers, B. P., Parks, M. H., Nickel, M. K., Katwal, S. B., & Martin, P. R. (2012). Reduced fronto-cerebellar functional connectivity in chronic alcoholic patients.* Alcoholism, Clinical and Experimental Research, 36*(2), 294–301. http://doi.org/10.1111/j.1530-0277.2011.01614.x.*

investigated the relationship between alcohol-dependence severity and FC of frontostriatal networks during response inhibition. Frontostriatal FC was assessed with a psychophysiological interaction analysis using the right putamen as a seed region to identify brain areas that correlated with activation in this region during successful performance on a stop-signal task. This analysis revealed that the right putamen showed significant connectivity (ie, positive correlation) with the subcallosal/anterior cingulate cortices and the paracingulate gyrus. Greater alcohol-dependence severity was associated with weaker FC between the putamen and prefrontal regions (eg, the anterior insula, anterior cingulate, and medial prefrontal cortex) during response inhibition. Reduced frontostriatal connectivity had been previously associated with failure to learn reward prediction errors (Parks et al., 2010). Such findings suggest an important role of this network in modulating impulsive behavior in AUD.

AUD seems to affect multiple cognitive, sensorimotor, and emotional processes and underlying brain networks. Müller-Oehring, Jung, Pfefferbaum, Sullivan, and Schulte (2015) investigated the integrity of multiple resting-state brain networks in AUD in relation to cognition and emotion. FC analysis assessed the DMN; in addition the EC, salience (SA), and attention (AT) networks; primary somatosensory, auditory, and visual (VI) input networks; and subcortical reward (RW) and emotion (EM) networks in 27 short-term abstinent men and 26 gender- and age-matched controls. The authors hypothesized that the different patterns of connectivity between alcoholics and controls could represent distinct neurobiological mechanisms, for example, (1) "network deficiency," that is, less or weaker connectivity in alcoholics relative to controls related to poor behavioral outcome; (2) "compensatory neural ability," that is, neural mechanisms to overcome processing deficiencies in the main nodes of the networks involving additional or stronger interregional connectivity in alcoholics relative to controls to achieve normal task performance; and (3) "network dedifferentiation," that is, when additional or stronger regional connectivity in alcoholics relative to controls is related to poor behavioral outcomes. The authors demonstrated that intrinsic connectivity in all examined brain networks was largely preserved in individuals with chronic alcoholism. Indeed, the two groups exhibited an extensive overlap of ongoing, intrinsic connectivity within these nine resting-state brain networks (Fig. 7), suggesting overall preserved integrity of large-scale functional systems in AUD. But despite this similar architecture, connectivity analyses identified specific lower intranetwork connectivity and, extensive connectivity to regions outside the main networks in alcoholics compared with controls, correlated with poor cognitive performance and altered mood. For DMN, SA, reward, and EC networks, both greater within-network and expanded outside-network connectivity correlated with poor performance and altered mood. Thus, it appears that alcoholics fail in confining "neural coherence" within these networks and recruit unnecessary nonspecialized regions outside these systems. That is to say, "they need more to do less." This evokes a form of functional network dedifferentiation in alcoholism (Schulte, Müller-Oehring, Rohlfing, Pfefferbaum, & Sullivan, 2010), similar to dedifferentiation

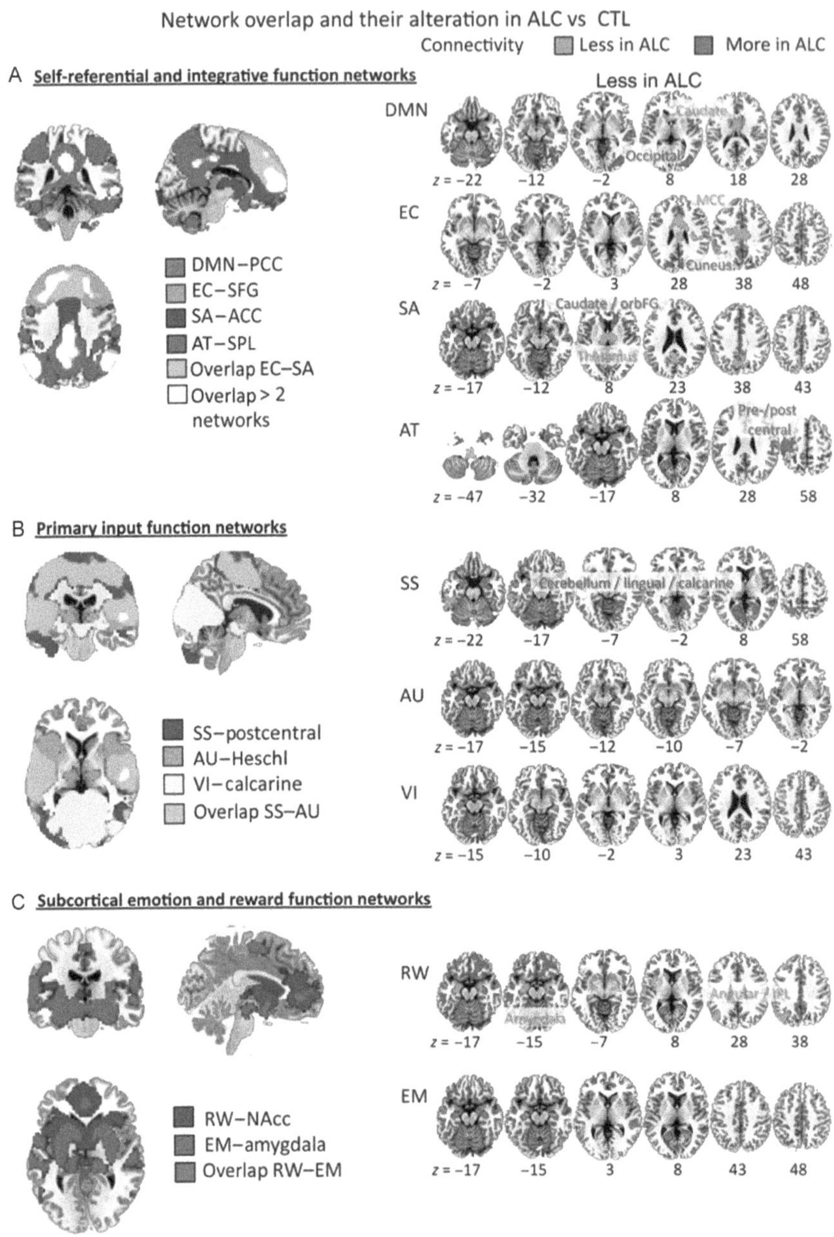

Fig. 7 Intrinsic network differences in alcoholics (ALC) relative to controls (CTL). *Left panels*: Illustration of network segregation and overlap for (A) self-referential (DMN–PCC seed) and integrative function networks (EC–SFG seed, SA–ACC seed, AT–SPL seed), (B) primary input function networks (SS–postcentral seed, AU–Heschl seed,

processes in aging that are marked by less distinctive activation patterns and less effective transfer of information between regions (Goh, 2011). By contrast, diffuse connectivity within attentional and visual networks in alcoholism was related to better task performance, strengthening the concept of increasing connectivity as a cerebral mechanism for functional compensation.

Concerning long-term abstinent alcoholics, it was observed that resting-state FC of the reward and EC networks (investigated using the nucleus accumbens and the subgenual cingulate cortex as seed voxels) differed in comparison to short-term abstinent alcoholic: resting-state synchrony within the reward network progressively decreased and in the EC network increased (Camchong, Stenger, & Fein, 2013). This suggests that during long abstinence, functional changes modify behaviors for sustaining abstinence. Furthermore, connectivity strength within the EC network was correlated with cognitive flexibility and connectivity strength within the reward network was correlated with the number of current antisocial symptoms in short-term abstinence. Findings of this study may reflect progressive adaptive mechanisms allowing abstinent alcoholics to inhibit and successfully stop behaviors that may lead to substance use.

Weiland et al. (2014) explored the association between alcohol use-related problems and resting-state FC in individuals ranging from binge drinkers to nonabstinent individuals with severe AUD. They chose to utilize 14 previously identified intrinsic connectivity networks (Shirer, Ryali, Rykhlevskaia, Menon, & Greicius, 2012) comprising a priori ROI that encompass the majority of the cortical and subcortical GM and can be mapped to common cognitive/motor functions (Fig. 8).

Fig. 7—cont'd VI–calcarine seed), and (C) subcortical emotion and reward networks (RW–NAcc seed, EM–amygdala seed). A result output image was created from group conjunction analysis for each seed's connectivity map with the same statistical threshold for all analyses (combined peak-and-extent threshold with peak $p < 0.001$ and extent $P_{FWE\text{-}corrected} < 0.05$). *Right panels*: For each network, illustration of altered seed-to-voxel connectivity in ALC relative to CTL: marked *red* (*gray* in the print version) when "expanded" and *green* (*light gray* in the print version) when "restricted" for masked contrast analysis; for group contrast analysis, regions are labeled in the figure and marked in *red* (*gray* in the print version) when ALC > CTL and *green* (*light gray* in the print version) when CTL > ALC; combined peak-and-extent threshold corrected for multiple comparisons $P_{FWE\text{-}corrected} < 0.05$. MNI *z*-coordinates indicate slice locations. *From Müller-Oehring, E. M., Jung, Y.-C., Pfefferbaum, A., Sullivan, E. V., & Schulte, T. (2015). The resting brain of alcoholics.* Cerebral Cortex (New York, N.Y.: 1991), *25(11), 4155–4168. http://doi.org/10.1093/cercor/bhu134.*

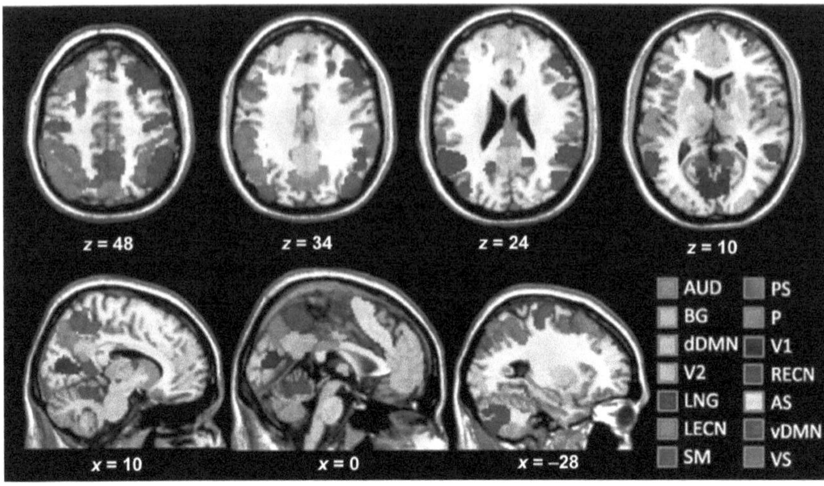

Fig. 8 Fourteen intrinsic connectivity networks. The ICNs are comprised of 90 distinct ROIs or nodes encompassing the majority of the cortical and subcortical gray matter that were downloaded from Stanford's FIND lab (Shirer et al., 2012) and include: auditory; primary and higher visual; language; sensorimotor; anterior and posterior salience; basal ganglia; dorsal, ventral, and precuneus default mode; and bilateral executive control systems. *From Weiland, B. J., Sabbineni, A., Calhoun, V. D., Welsh, R. C., Bryan, A. D., Jung, R. E., … Hutchison, K. E. (2014). Reduced left executive control network functional connectivity is associated with alcohol use disorders.* Alcoholism, Clinical and Experimental Research, *38(9), 2445–2453. http://doi.org/10.1111/acer.12505.*

Analyses tested for differences in network connectivity strength, a global measure of connectivity calculated as the mean of all pairwise correlations between nodes within each network (Lynall et al., 2010). They showed that individuals with severe AUD had significantly lower network connectivity strength than controls in the left EC, basal ganglia, sensorimotor, and primary visual networks (Fig. 9).

Further, for the entire sample of individuals with severe AUD, left EC network connectivity strength was negatively associated with measures of hazardous drinking and loss of control over alcohol consumption. Within this network, they identified key nodes significantly associated with disease severity. They found negative correlations between impaired behavioral control and scores on the AUDIT (Alcohol Use Disorders Identification Test; Saunders et al., 1993) and connectivity between the parietal, dorsal lateral prefrontal cortex, middle frontal gyrus, and caudate nodes suggesting dysfunction of this network. These results are consistent with studies that have reported negative associations between WM integrity tracts linking frontal and parietal regions and substance use (Pfefferbaum et al., 2009; Schulte et al., 2010).

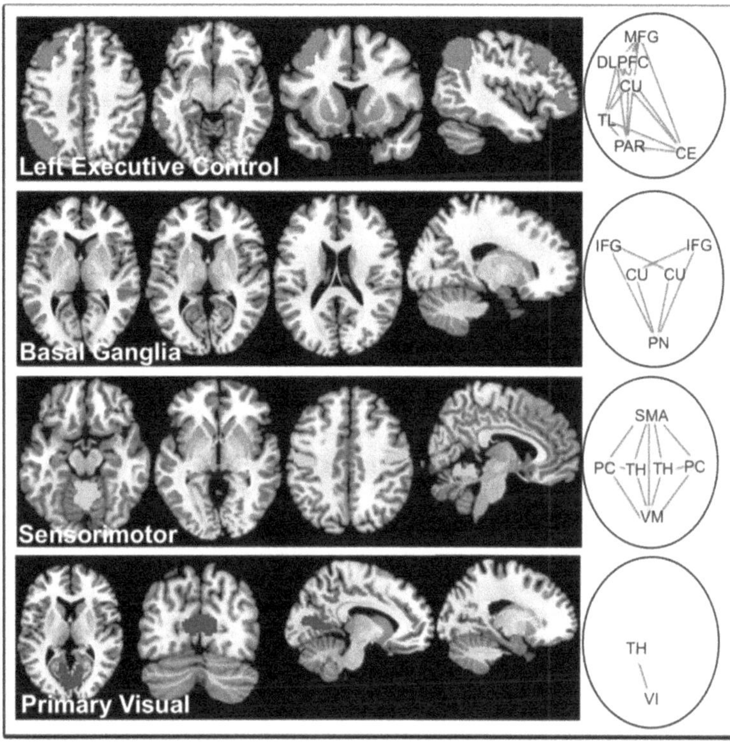

Fig. 9 Networks different between ALC subjects and controls ROIs defining the networks with significantly lower connectivity strength in age- and gender-matched ALC subjects ($n = 255$) and controls ($n = 87$) include the left executive control (LECN), basal ganglia (BG), sensorimotor (SM), and primary visual (PV) network's. *From Weiland, B. J., Sabbineni, A., Calhoun, V. D., Welsh, R. C., Bryan, A. D., Jung, R. E., … Hutchison, K. E. (2014). Reduced left executive control network functional connectivity is associated with alcohol use disorders.* Alcoholism, Clinical and Experimental Research, *38(9), 2445–2453. http://doi.org/10.1111/acer.12505.*

All these findings indicate that AUD negatively impacts brain connectivity, specifically in the EC network. Altered FC in this specific network may represent an underlying mechanism for control dysfunction and contribute to inability to restrain alcohol consumption. Indeed, dorsal lateral prefrontal cortex and middle frontal gyrus are two key nodes of this network showing poor basal functioning; they are thought to be involved in top-down attentional focus and emotional processing (mood awareness and regulation), respectively. Thus, lower FC between these key regions potentially contributes to poor behavioral control.

4. CONCLUSION

AUD is unfortunately a very common disorder, affecting people of all ages and socioeconomic groups. It may cause serious damage to major aspects of an individual's life as well as society as a whole. Thus, treatment and prevention of AUD is a major public health concern. To reduce AUD incidence, it is essential to better understand this complex disorder. A better understanding of AUD requires the consideration of multiple aspects, the participation of several disciplines, and the use of many resources. Neuroimaging is a powerful means to investigate the brain correlates of AUD. Multimodal imaging is necessary because no single imaging methodology can elucidate all relevant characteristics of AUD (Schulte et al., 2012). The MRI studies reported here have revealed that AUD is associated with structural and functional brain alterations. Structural brain imaging provides evidence for cortical shrinkage and extensive GM and WM volume loss in alcoholism, with considerable vulnerability found in frontocerebellar brain circuit. Functional MRI has revealed AUD-related alterations in brain activity during performance of wide variety of tasks. Overall, fMRI findings are consistent with structural data and indicate that frontal brain systems are particularly vulnerable. Resting-state fMRI results converge to support dysfunctional connectivity with the executive control network appearing to be particularly damaged in AUD. Such brain alterations seem to affect multiple cognitive, sensorimotor, and emotional processes.

REFERENCES

Agartz, I., Momenan, R., Rawlings, R. R., Kerich, M. J., & Hommer, D. W. (1999). Hippocampal volume in patients with alcohol dependence. *Archives of General Psychiatry*, *56*(4), 356–363.

Allen, E. A., Erhardt, E. B., Damaraju, E., Gruner, W., Segall, J. M., Silva, R. F., … Calhoun, V. D. (2011). A baseline for the multivariate comparison of resting-state networks. *Frontiers in Systems Neuroscience*, *5*, 2. http://doi.org/10.3389/fnsys.2011.00002.

American Psychiatric Association (2000). *Diagnostic and statistical manual of mental disorders* (4th ed., text rev., pp. 191–296). Arlington, VA: American Psychiatric Publishing.

American Psychiatric Association (2013). *Diagnostic and statistical manual of mental disorders* (5th ed., pp. 481–590). Arlington, VA: American Psychiatric Publishing.

Andrews-Hanna, J. R., Snyder, A. Z., Vincent, J. L., Lustig, C., Head, D., Raichle, M. E., & Buckner, R. L. (2007). Disruption of large-scale brain systems in advanced aging. *Neuron*, *56*(5), 924–935. http://doi.org/10.1016/j.neuron.2007.10.038.

Antunez, E., Estruch, R., Cardenal, C., Nicolas, J. M., Fernandez-Sola, J., & Urbano-Marquez, A. (1998). Usefulness of CT and MR imaging in the diagnosis of acute Wernicke's encephalopathy. *AJR American Journal of Roentgenology*, *171*(4), 1131–1137. http://doi.org/10.2214/ajr.171.4.9763009.

Ashburner, J., & Friston, K. J. (2000). Voxel-based morphometry—The methods. *NeuroImage, 11*(6 Pt. 1), 805–821. http://doi.org/10.1006/nimg.2000.0582.

Balsters, J. H., & Ramnani, N. (2011). Cerebellar plasticity and the automation of first-order rules. *The Journal of Neuroscience: The Official Journal of the Society for Neuroscience, 31*(6), 2305–2312. http://doi.org/10.1523/JNEUROSCI.4358-10.2011.

Balsters, J. H., Whelan, C. D., Robertson, I. H., & Ramnani, N. (2013). Cerebellum and cognition: Evidence for the encoding of higher order rules. *Cerebral Cortex (New York, N.Y. 1991), 23*(6), 1433–1443. http://doi.org/10.1093/cercor/bhs127.

Beckmann, C. F., DeLuca, M., Devlin, J. T., & Smith, S. M. (2005). Investigations into resting-state connectivity using independent component analysis. *Philosophical Transactions: Biological Sciences, 360*(1457), 1001.

Beresford, T., Arciniegas, D., Alters, J., Clapp, L., Martin, B., Du, Y., & Davatzikos, C. (2006). Hippocampus volume loss due to chronic heavy drinking (English). *Alcoholism, Clinical and Experimental Research, 30*(11), 1866–1870.

Biswal, B., Yetkin, F. Z., Haughton, V. M., & Hyde, J. S. (1995). Functional connectivity in the motor cortex of resting human brain using echo-planar MRI. *Magnetic Resonance in Medicine, 34*, 537–541.

Bleich, S., Sperling, W., Degner, D., Graesel, E., Bleich, K., Wilhelm, J., ... Kornhuber, J. (2003). Lack of association between hippocampal volume reduction and first-onset alcohol withdrawal seizure. A volumetric MRI study. *Alcohol and Alcoholism (Oxford, Oxfordshire), 38*(1), 40–44.

Bloomer, C. W., Langleben, D. D., & Meyerhoff, D. J. (2004). Magnetic resonance detects brainstem changes in chronic, active heavy drinkers. *Psychiatry Research, 132*(3), 209–218. http://doi.org/10.1016/j.pscychresns.2004.06.003.

Bouchery, E. E., Harwood, H. J., Sacks, J. J., Simon, C. J., & Brewer, R. D. (2011). Economic costs of excessive alcohol consumption in the U.S., 2006. *American Journal of Preventive Medicine, 41*(5), 516–524. http://doi.org/10.1016/j.amepre.2011.06.045.

Boutte, D., Calhoun, V. D., Chen, J., Sabbineni, A., Hutchison, K., & Liu, J. (2012). Association of genetic copy number variations at 11 q14.2 with brain regional volume differences in an alcohol use disorder population. *Alcohol (Fayetteville, NY), 46*(6), 519–527. http://dx.doi.org/10.1016/j.alcohol.2012.05.002.

Buckner, R. L., Andrews-Hanna, J. R., & Schacter, D. L. (2008a). The brain's default network: Anatomy, function, and relevance to disease. In A. Kingstone, M. B. Miller, A. Kingstone, & M. B. Miller (Eds.), *The year in cognitive neuroscience 2008* (pp. 1–38). Malden: Blackwell Publishing.

Buckner, R. L., Andrews-Hanna, J. R., & Schacter, D. L. (2008b). The brain's default network: Anatomy, function, and relevance to disease. *Annals of the New York Academy of Sciences, 1124*, 1–38. http://doi.org/10.1196/annals.1440.011.

Camchong, J., Stenger, V. A., & Fein, G. (2013). Resting-state synchrony in short-term versus long-term abstinent alcoholics. *Alcoholism, Clinical and Experimental Research, 37*(5), 794–803. http://doi.org/10.1111/acer.12037.

Cardenas, V. A., Studholme, C., Gazdzinski, S., Durazzo, T. C., & Meyerhoff, D. J. (2007). Deformation-based morphometry of brain changes in alcohol dependence and abstinence. *NeuroImage, 34*, 879–887. http://dx.doi.org/10.1016/j.neuroimage.2006.10.015.

Chanraud, S., Martelli, C., Delain, F., Kostogianni, N., Douaud, G., Aubin, H., ... Martinot, J. (2007). Brain morphometry and cognitive performance in detoxified alcohol-dependents with preserved psychosocial functioning. *Neuropsychopharmacology: Official Publication of the American College of Neuropsychopharmacology, 32*(2), 429–438. http://doi.org/10.1038/sj.npp.1301219.

Chanraud, S., Pitel, A.-L., Müller-Oehring, E. M., Pfefferbaum, A., & Sullivan, E. V. (2013). Remapping the brain to compensate for impairment in recovering alcoholics. *Cerebral Cortex (New York, N.Y. 1991), 23*(1), 97–104. http://doi.org/10.1093/cercor/bhr381.

Chanraud, S., Pitel, A.-L., Pfefferbaum, A., & Sullivan, E. V. (2011). Disruption of functional connectivity of the default-mode network in alcoholism. *Cerebral Cortex (New York, N.Y. 1991)*, *21*(10), 2272–2281. http://doi.org/10.1093/cercor/bhq297.
Chanraud, S., Reynaud, M., Wessa, M., Penttilä, J., Kostogianni, N., Cachia, A., … Martinot, J.-L. (2009). Diffusion tensor tractography in mesencephalic bundles: Relation to mental flexibility in detoxified alcohol-dependent subjects. *Neuropsychopharmacology: Official Publication of the American College of Neuropsychopharmacology*, *34*(5), 1223–1232. http://doi.org/10.1038/npp.2008.101.
Chanraud, S., Zahr, N., Sullivan, E. V., & Pfefferbaum, A. (2010). MR diffusion tensor imaging: A window into white matter integrity of the working brain. *Neuropsychology Review*, *20*(2), 209–225. http://doi.org/10.1007/s11065-010-9129-7.
Clark, D. B., Thatcher, D. L., & Tapert, S. F. (2008). Alcohol, psychological dysregulation, and adolescent brain development. *Alcoholism, Clinical and Experimental Research*, *32*(3), 375–385. http://dx.doi.org/10.1111/j.1530-0277.2007.00601.x.
Courtney, K. E., Ghahremani, D. G., & Ray, L. A. (2013). Fronto-striatal functional connectivity during response inhibition in alcohol dependence. *Addiction Biology*, *18*(3), 593–604. http://doi.org/10.1111/adb.12013.
Davis, S. W., Dennis, N. A., Daselaar, S. M., Fleck, M. S., & Cabeza, R. (2008). Que PASA? The posterior-anterior shift in aging. *Cerebral Cortex*, *18*(5), 1201–1209. http://doi.org/10.1093/cercor/bhm155.
Desmond, J. E., Chen, S. H. A., DeRosa, E., Pryor, M. R., Pfefferbaum, A., & Sullivan, E. V. (2003). Increased frontocerebellar activation in alcoholics during verbal working memory: An fMRI study. *NeuroImage*, *19*(4), 1510–1520.
Durkee, C. A., Sarlls, J. E., Hommer, D. W., & Momenan, R. (2013). White matter microstructure alterations: A study of alcoholics with and without post-traumatic stress disorder. *PloS One*, *8*(11), e80952. http://doi.org/10.1371/journal.pone.0080952.
Estruch, R., Nicolás, J. M., Salamero, M., Aragón, C., Sacanella, E., Fernández-Solà, J., & Urbano-Márquez, A. (1997). Atrophy of the corpus callosum in chronic alcoholism. *Journal of the Neurological Sciences*, *146*(2), 145–151.
Fein, G., Landman, B., Tran, H., McGillivray, S., Finn, P., Barakos, J., & Moon, K. (2006). Brain atrophy in long-term abstinent alcoholics who demonstrate impairment on a simulated gambling task. *NeuroImage*, *32*, 1465–1471. http://dx.doi.org/10.1016/j.neuroimage.2006.06.013.
Ferreira, L. K., & Busatto, G. F. (2013). Review: Resting-state functional connectivity in normal brain aging. *Neuroscience and Biobehavioral Reviews*, *37*, 384–400. http://dx.doi.org/10.1016/j.neubiorev.2013.01.017.
Fortier, C. B., Leritz, E. C., Salat, D. H., Venne, J. R., Maksimovskiy, A. L., Williams, V., & McGlinchey, R. E. (2011). Reduced cortical thickness in abstinent alcoholics and association with alcoholic behavior. *Alcoholism, Clinical and Experimental Research*, *35*(12), 2193–2201.
Fox, M. D., & Raichle, M. E. (2007). Spontaneous fluctuations in brain activity observed with functional magnetic resonance imaging. *Nature Reviews. Neuroscience*, *8*(9), 700–711.
Gazdzinski, S., Durazzo, T. C., Weiner, M. W., & Meyerhoff, D. J. (2008). Are treated alcoholics representative of the entire population with alcohol use disorders? A magnetic resonance study of brain injury. *Alcohol (Fayetteville, N.Y.)*, *42*(2), 67–76. http://doi.org/10.1016/j.alcohol.2008.01.002.
Geschwind, N. (2010). Disconnexion syndromes in animals and man: Part I. 1965. *Neuropsychology Review*, *20*(2), 128–157.
Gilman, J. M., Davis, M. B., & Hommer, D. W. (2010). Greater activation in left hemisphere language-related regions during simple judgment tasks among substance-dependent patients in treatment for alcoholism. *Alcoholism, Clinical and Experimental Research*, *34*(2), 331–341. http://doi.org/10.1111/j.1530-0277.2009.01095.x.

Goh, J. O. S. (2011). Functional dedifferentiation and altered connectivity in older adults: Neural accounts of cognitive aging. *Aging and Disease*, *2*(1), 30–48.

Grodin, E. N., Lin, H., Durkee, C. A., Hommer, D. W., & Momenan, R. (2013). Deficits in cortical, diencephalic and midbrain gray matter in alcoholism measured by VBM: Effects of co-morbid substance abuse. *NeuroImage Clinical*, *2*, 469–476. http://dx.doi.org/10.1016/j.nicl.2013.03.013.

Harding, A. J., Wong, A., Svoboda, M., Kril, J. J., & Halliday, G. M. (1997). Chronic alcohol consumption does not cause hippocampal neuron loss in humans. *Hippocampus*, 7(1), 78–87. http://doi.org/10.1002/(SICI)1098-1063(1997)7:13.0.CO;2-3.

Harper, C. (1998). The neuropathology of alcohol-specific brain damage, or does alcohol damage the brain? *Journal of Neuropathology and Experimental Neurology*, *57*(2), 101–110.

Harper, C., & Matsumoto, I. (2005). Ethanol and brain damage. *Current Opinion in Pharmacology*, *5*, 73–78. http://dx.doi.org/10.1016/j.coph.2004.06.011.

Harris, G. J., Jaffin, S. K., Hodge, S. M., Kennedy, D., Caviness, V. S., Marinkovic, K., … Oscar-Berman, M. (2008). Frontal white matter and cingulum diffusion tensor imaging deficits in alcoholism. *Alcoholism, Clinical and Experimental Research*, *32*(6), 1001–1013. http://doi.org/10.1111/j.1530-0277.2008.00661.x.

He, D. Y., McGough, N. N. H., Ravindranathan, A., Jeanblanc, J., Logrip, M. L., Phamluong, K., & Ron, D. (2005). Glial cell line-derived neurotrophic factor mediates the desirable actions of the anti-addiction drug ibogaine against alcohol consumption. *The Journal of Neuroscience: The Official Journal of the Society for Neuroscience*, *25*(3), 619–628. http://doi.org/10.1523/JNEUROSCI.3959-04.2005.

Jones, D. K., Knösche, T. R., & Turner, R. (2013). White matter integrity, fiber count, and other fallacies: The do's and don'ts of diffusion MRI. *NeuroImage*, *73*, 239–254. http://doi.org/10.1016/j.neuroimage.2012.06.081.

Jung, Y. C., Jang, D.-P., Namkoong, K., Ku, J., Kim, J.-J., Park, S., … Lee, E. (2007). Shape deformation of the insula in alcoholics: Reduction of left-right asymmetry. *Neuroreport*, *18*(17), 1787–1791. http://doi.org/10.1097/WNR.0b013e3282f193b4.

Kamarajan, C., Porjesz, B., Jones, K., Chorlian, D., Padmanabhapillai, A., Rangaswamy, M., … Begleiter, H. (2006). Event-related oscillations in offspring of alcoholics: Neurocognitive disinhibition as a risk for alcoholism. *Biological Psychiatry*, *59*(7), 625–634. http://doi.org/10.1016/j.biopsych.2005.08.017.

Kurth, C., Wegerer, V., Reulbach, U., Lewczuk, P., Kornhuber, J., Steinhoff, B. J., & Bleich, S. (2004). Analysis of hippocampal atrophy in alcoholic patients by a Kohonen feature map. *Neuroreport*, *15*(2), 367–371.

Laakso, M., Vaurio, O., Savolainen, L., Repo, E., Soininen, H., Aronen, H., & Tiihonen, J. (2000). A volumetric MRI study of the hippocampus in type 1 and 2 alcoholism. *Behavioural Brain Research*, *109*(2), 177.

Lander, L., Howsare, J., & Byrne, M. (2013). The impact of substance use disorders on families and children: From theory to practice. *Social Work in Public Health*, *28*(3–4), 194–205. http://doi.org/10.1080/19371918.2013.759005.

Lipton, S. A., Kim, W., Choi, Y., Kumar, S., D'Emilia, D. M., Rayudu, P. V., … Stamler, J. S. (1997). Neurotoxicity associated with dual actions of homocysteine at the *N*-methyl-D-aspartate receptor. *Proceedings of the National Academy of Sciences of the United States of America*, *94*(11), 5923.

Lynall, M.-E., Bassett, D. S., Kerwin, R., McKenna, P. J., Kitzbichler, M., Muller, U., & Bullmore, E. (2010). Functional connectivity and brain networks in schizophrenia. *Journal of Neuroscience*, *30*(28), 9477–9487. http://doi.org/10.1523/JNEUROSCI.0333-10.2010.

Makris, N., Oscar-Berman, M., Jaffin, S. K., Hodge, S. M., Kennedy, D. N., Caviness, V. S., … Harris, G. J. (2008). Decreased volume of the brain reward system in alcoholism. *Biological Psychiatry*, *64*(3), 192–202. http://dx.doi.org/10.1016/j.biopsych.2008.01.018.

Mann, K., Schäfer, D. R., Längle, G., Ackermann, K., & Croissant, B. (2005). The long-term course of alcoholism, 5, 10 and 16 years after treatment. *Addiction (Abingdon, England)*, *100*(6), 797–805. http://doi.org/10.1111/j.1360-0443.2005.01065.x.

Margulies, D. S., Vincent, J. L., Kelly, C., Lohmann, G., Uddin, L. Q., Biswal, B. B., … Petrides, M. (2009). Precuneus shares intrinsic functional architecture in humans and monkeys. *Proceedings of the National Academy of Sciences of the United States of America*, *106*(47), 20069.

Marinkovic, K., Oscar-Berman, M., Urban, T., O'Reilly, C. E., Howard, J. A., Sawyer, K., & Harris, G. J. (2009). Alcoholism and dampened temporal limbic activation to emotional faces. *Alcoholism, Clinical and Experimental Research*, *33*(11), 1880–1892. http://doi.org/10.1111/j.1530-0277.2009.01026.x.

Marrelec, G., & Fransson, P. (2011). Assessing the influence of different ROI selection strategies on functional connectivity analyses of fMRI data acquired during steady-state conditions. *PloS One*, *6*(4), e14788. http://doi.org/10.1371/journal.pone.0014788.

Marshall, E. J., & Farrell, M. (2007). Substance use and psychiatric comorbidity. *Medicine*, *35*(4), 246–249. http://doi.org/10.1016/j.mpmed.2007.02.010.

McBride, W. J. (2002). Central nucleus of the amygdala and the effects of alcohol and alcohol-drinking behavior in rodents. *Pharmacology, Biochemistry and Behavior*, *71*, 509–515. http://dx.doi.org/10.1016/S0091-3057(01)00680-3 (Functional role of specific systems within the extended amygdala and hypothalamus).

Mechtcheriakov, S., Brenneis, C., Egger, K., Koppelstaetter, F., Schocke, M., & Marksteiner, J. (2007). A widespread distinct pattern of cerebral atrophy in patients with alcohol addiction revealed by voxel-based morphometry. *Journal of Neurology, Neurosurgery and Psychiatry*, *78*(6), 610.

Monnig, M. A., Caprihan, A., Yeo, R. A., Gasparovic, C., Ruhl, D. A., Lysne, P., … Thoma, R. J. (2013). Diffusion tensor imaging of white matter networks in individuals with current and remitted alcohol use disorders and comorbid conditions. *Psychology of Addictive Behaviors*, *27*(2), 455–465. http://doi.org/10.1037/a0027168.

Monnig, M. A., Yeo, R. A., Tonigan, J. S., McCrady, B. S., Thoma, R. J., Sabbineni, A., & Hutchison, K. E. (2015). Associations of white matter microstructure with clinical and demographic characteristics in heavy drinkers. *PloS One*, *10*(11), e0142042. http://doi.org/10.1371/journal.pone.0142042.

Moselhy, H. F., Georgiou, G., & Kahn, A. (2001). Frontal lobe changes in alcoholism: A review of the literature. *Alcohol and Alcoholism (Oxford, Oxfordshire)*, *36*(5), 357–368. http://dx.doi.org/10.1093/alcalc/36.5.357.

Müller-Oehring, E. M., Jung, Y.-C., Pfefferbaum, A., Sullivan, E. V., & Schulte, T. (2015). The resting brain of alcoholics. *Cerebral Cortex (New York, N.Y. 1991)*, *25*(11), 4155–4168. http://doi.org/10.1093/cercor/bhu134.

Müller-Oehring, E. M., Schulte, T., Fama, R., Pfefferbaum, A., & Sullivan, E. V. (2009). Global-local interference is related to callosal compromise in alcoholism: A behavior-DTI association study. *Alcoholism, Clinical and Experimental Research*, *33*(3), 477–489. http://doi.org/10.1111/j.1530-0277.2008.00858.x.

Nixon, K., & Crews, F. T. (2004). Temporally specific burst in cell proliferation increases hippocampal neurogenesis in protracted abstinence from alcohol. *The Journal of Neuroscience: The Official Journal of the Society for Neuroscience*, *24*(43), 9714–9722. http://doi.org/10.1523/JNEUROSCI.3063-04.2004.

Norris, D. G. (2006). Principles of magnetic resonance assessment of brain function. *Journal of Magnetic Resonance Imaging: JMRI*, *23*(6), 794–807. http://doi.org/10.1002/jmri.20587.

Parks, M. H., Greenberg, D. S., Nickel, M. K., Dietrich, M. S., Rogers, B. P., & Martin, P. R. (2010). Recruitment of additional brain regions to accomplish simple motor tasks in chronic alcohol-dependent patients. *Alcoholism, Clinical and Experimental Research*, *34*(6), 1098–1109. http://doi.org/10.1111/j.1530-0277.2010.01186.x.

Pfefferbaum, A., Adalsteinsson, E., & Sullivan, E. V. (2005). Frontal circuitry degradation marks healthy adult aging: Evidence from diffusion tensor imaging. *NeuroImage, 26*(3), 891–899. http://doi.org/10.1016/j.neuroimage.2005.02.034.

Pfefferbaum, A., Adalsteinsson, E., & Sullivan, E. V. (2006). Dysmorphology and microstructural degradation of the corpus callosum: Interaction of age and alcoholism. *Neurobiology of Aging, 27*(7), 994–1009. http://doi.org/10.1016/j.neurobiolaging.2005.05.007.

Pfefferbaum, A., Desmond, J. E., Galloway, C., Menon, V., Glover, G. H., & Sullivan, E. V. (2001). Reorganization of frontal systems used by alcoholics for spatial working memory: An fMRI study. *NeuroImage, 14*(1 Pt. 1), 7–20. http://doi.org/10.1006/nimg.2001.0785.

Pfefferbaum, A., Lim, K. O., Desmond, J. E., & Sullivan, E. V. (1996). Thinning of the corpus callosum in older alcoholic men: A magnetic resonance imaging study. *Alcoholism, Clinical and Experimental Research, 20*(4), 752–757.

Pfefferbaum, A., Rosenbloom, M., Deshmukh, A., & Sullivan, E. (2001). Sex differences in the effects of alcohol on brain structure. *The American Journal of Psychiatry, 158*(2), 188–197. http://doi.org/10.1176/appi.ajp.158.2.188.

Pfefferbaum, A., Rosenbloom, M. J., Fama, R., Sassoon, S. A., & Sullivan, E. V. (2010). Transcallosal white matter degradation detected with quantitative fiber tracking in alcoholic men and women: Selective relations to dissociable functions. *Alcoholism, Clinical and Experimental Research, 34*(7), 1201–1211. http://doi.org/10.1111/j.1530-0277.2010.01197.x.

Pfefferbaum, A., Rosenbloom, M., Rohlfing, T., & Sullivan, E. V. (2009). Degradation of association and projection white matter systems in alcoholism detected with quantitative fiber tracking. *Biological Psychiatry, 65*(8), 680–690. http://doi.org/10.1016/j.biopsych.2008.10.039.

Pfefferbaum, A., Rosenbloom, M., Serventi, K. L., & Sullivan, E. V. (2002). Corpus callosum, pons, and cortical white matter in alcoholic women. *Alcoholism, Clinical and Experimental Research, 26*(3), 400–406.

Pfefferbaum, A., Sullivan, E. V., Hedehus, M., Adalsteinsson, E., Lim, K. O., & Moseley, M. (2000). In vivo detection and functional correlates of white matter microstructural disruption in chronic alcoholism. *Alcoholism, Clinical and Experimental Research, 24*(8), 1214–1221.

Raichle, M. E., MacLeod, A. M., Snyder, A. Z., Powers, W. J., Gusnard, D. A., & Shulman, G. L. (2001). A default mode of brain function. *Proceedings of the National Academy of Sciences of the United States of America, 98*(2), 676. http://doi.org/10.1073/pnas.98.2.676.

Raichle, M. E., & Mintun, M. A. (2006). Brain work and brain imaging. *Annual Review of Neuroscience, 29*, 449–476. http://doi.org/10.1146/annurev.neuro.29.051605.112819.

Raichle, M. E., & Snyder, A. Z. (2007). A default mode of brain function: A brief history of an evolving idea. *NeuroImage, 37*(4), 1083–1090. discussion 1097–1099, http://doi.org/10.1016/j.neuroimage.2007.02.041.

Rando, K., Kwang-Ik, H., Bhagwagar, Z., Chiang-Shan Ray, L., Bergquist, K., Guarnaccia, J., & Sinha, R. (2011). Association of frontal and posterior cortical gray matter volume with time to alcohol relapse: A prospective study. *American Journal of Psychiatry, 168*(2), 183.

Rogers, B. P., Parks, M. H., Nickel, M. K., Katwal, S. B., & Martin, P. R. (2012). Reduced fronto-cerebellar functional connectivity in chronic alcoholic patients. *Alcoholism, Clinical and Experimental Research, 36*(2), 294–301. http://doi.org/10.1111/j.1530-0277.2011.01614.x.

Ruiz, S. M., Oscar-Berman, M., Sawyer, K. S., Valmas, M. M., Urban, T., & Harris, G. J. (2013). Drinking history associations with regional white matter volumes in alcoholic men and women. *Alcoholism, Clinical and Experimental Research, 37*(1), 110–122. http://dx.doi.org/10.1111/j.1530-0277.2012.01862.

Saunders, J. B., Aasland, O. G., Babor, T. F., de la Fuente, J. R., & Grant, M. (1993). Development of the alcohol use disorders identification test (AUDIT): WHO collaborative project on early detection of persons with harmful alcohol consumption—II. *Addiction (Abingdon, England)*, *88*(6), 791–804.

Schmahmann, J. D., & Pandya, D. N. (1997). The cerebrocerebellar system. *International Review of Neurobiology*, *41*, 31–60.

Schulte, T., Müller-Oehring, E. M., Rohlfing, T., Pfefferbaum, A., & Sullivan, E. V. (2010). White matter fiber degradation attenuates hemispheric asymmetry when integrating visuomotor information. *The Journal of Neuroscience: The Official Journal of the Society for Neuroscience*, *30*(36), 12168–12178. http://doi.org/10.1523/JNEUROSCI.2160-10.2010.

Schulte, T., Müller-Oehring, E. M., Sullivan, E. V., & Pfefferbaum, A. (2012). Synchrony of corticostriatal-midbrain activation enables normal inhibitory control and conflict processing in recovering alcoholic men. *Biological Psychiatry*, *71*(3), 269–278. http://doi.org/10.1016/j.biopsych.2011.10.022.

Schulte, T., Oberlin, B. G., Kareken, D. A., Marinkovic, K., Müller-Oehring, E. M., Meyerhoff, D. J., & Tapert, S. (2012). How acute and chronic alcohol consumption affects brain networks: Insights from multimodal neuroimaging. *Alcoholism: Clinical and Experimental Research*, *36*(12), 2017–2027. http://doi.org/10.1111/j.1530-0277.2012.01831.x.

Shirer, W. R., Ryali, S., Rykhlevskaia, E., Menon, V., & Greicius, M. D. (2012). Decoding subject-driven cognitive states with whole-brain connectivity patterns. *Cerebral Cortex*, *22*(1), 158–165. http://doi.org/10.1093/cercor/bhr099.

Shulman, G. L., Fiez, J. A., Corbetta, M., Buckner, R. L., Miezin, F. M., Raichle, M. E., & Petersen, S. E. (1997). Common blood flow changes across visual tasks: II. Decreases in cerebral cortex. *Journal of Cognitive Neuroscience*, *9*(5), 648–663. http://doi.org/10.1162/jocn.1997.9.5.648.

Singh, V., Epstein-Ngo, Q., Cunningham, R. M., Stoddard, S. A., Chermack, S. T., & Walton, M. A. (2015). Physical dating violence among adolescents and young adults with alcohol misuse. *Drug and Alcohol Dependence*, *153*, 364–368. http://doi.org/10.1016/j.drugalcdep.2015.05.003.

Sullivan, E. V., Deshmukh, A., De Rosa, E., Rosenbloom, M. J., & Pfefferbaum, A. (2005). Striatal and forebrain nuclei volumes: Contribution to motor function and working memory deficits in alcoholism. *Biological Psychiatry*, *57*, 768–776. http://dx.doi.org/10.1016/j.biopsych.2004.12.012.

Sullivan, E. V., Deshmukh, A., Desmond, J. E., Lim, K. O., & Pfefferbaum, A. (2000). Cerebellar volume decline in normal aging, alcoholism, and Korsakoff's syndrome: Relation to ataxia. *Neuropsychology*, *14*(3), 341–352.

Sullivan, E., & Marsh, L. (2003). Hippocampal volume deficits in alcoholic Korsakoff's syndrome (English). *Neurology*, *61*(12), 1716–1719.

Sullivan, E. V., Marsh, L., Mathalon, D. H., Lim, K. O., & Pfefferbaum, A. (1995). Anterior hippocampal volume deficits in nonamnesic, aging chronic alcoholics. *Alcoholism, Clinical and Experimental Research*, *19*(1), 110–122. http://dx.doi.org/10.1111/j.1530-0277.1995.tb01478.x.

Tapert, S. F., Brown, G. G., Kindermann, S. S., Cheung, E. H., Frank, L. R., & Brown, S. A. (2001). fMRI measurement of brain dysfunction in alcohol-dependent young women. *Alcoholism, Clinical and Experimental Research*, *25*(2), 236–245.

Tessner, K. D., & Hill, S. Y. (2010). Neural circuitry associated with risk for alcohol use disorders. *Neuropsychology Review*, *20*(1), 1–20. http://doi.org/10.1007/s11065-009-9111-4.

Weiland, B. J., Sabbineni, A., Calhoun, V. D., Welsh, R. C., Bryan, A. D., Jung, R. E., ... Hutchison, K. E. (2014). Reduced left executive control network functional connectivity is associated with alcohol use disorders. *Alcoholism, Clinical and Experimental Research*, *38*(9), 2445–2453. http://doi.org/10.1111/acer.12505.

Wilhelm, J., Frieling, H., Hillemacher, T., Degner, D., Kornhuber, J., & Bleich, S. (2008). Hippocampal volume loss in patients with alcoholism is influenced by the consumed type of alcoholic beverage. *Alcohol and Alcoholism (Oxford, Oxfordshire)*, *43*(3), 296–299.

World Health Organization (2010). *Atlas on substance use: Resources for the prevention and treatment of substance use disorders*. Retrieved from, http://www.who.int/gho/substance_abuse/en/.

World Health Organization (2011). *Global status report on alcohol and health*. Retrieved from, http://www.who.int/substance_abuse/publications/global_alcohol_report/msbgsruprofiles.pdf?ua=1.

World Health Organization (2014). *Prevalence of alcohol use disorders*. Retrieved from, http://www.who.int/gho/substance_abuse/burden/alcohol_prevalence/en/.

Wrase, J., Makris, N., Braus, D. F., Mann, K., Smolka, M. N., Kennedy, D. N., … Heinz, A. (2008). Amygdala volume associated with alcohol abuse relapse and craving. *American Journal of Psychiatry*, *165*(9), 1179–1184. http://doi.org/10.1176/appi.ajp.2008.07121877.

Yeh, P.-H., Simpson, K., Durazzo, T. C., Gazdzinski, S., & Meyerhoff, D. J. (2009). Tract-based spatial statistics (TBSS) of diffusion tensor imaging data in alcohol dependence: Abnormalities of the motivational neurocircuitry. *Psychiatry Research*, *173*(1), 22–30. http://doi.org/10.1016/j.pscychresns.2008.07.012.

Zahr, N. M. (2014). Structural and microstructural imaging of the brain in alcohol use disorders. *Handbook of Clinical Neurology*, *125*, 275–290. http://doi.org/10.1016/B978-0-444-62619-6.00017-3.

Zahr, N. M., Pitel, A.-L., Chanraud, S., & Sullivan, E. V. (2010). Contributions of studies on alcohol use disorders to understanding cerebellar function. *Neuropsychology Review*, *20*(3), 280–289. http://doi.org/10.1007/s11065-010-9141-y.

CHAPTER TWO

Effects of Marijuana Use on Brain Structure and Function: Neuroimaging Findings from a Neurodevelopmental Perspective

T. Brumback[*,†,1], N. Castro[*], J. Jacobus[*,†], S. Tapert[*]
[*]University of California, San Diego, La Jolla, CA, United States
[†]VA San Diego Healthcare System, San Diego, CA, United States
[1]Corresponding author: e-mail address: tbrumback@ucsd.edu

Contents

Abstract

Marijuana, behind only tobacco and alcohol, is the most popular recreational drug in America with prevalence rates of use rising over the past decade. A wide range of research has highlighted neurocognitive deficits associated with marijuana use, particularly when initiated during childhood or adolescence. Neuroimaging, describing alterations to brain structure and function, has begun to provide a picture of possible mechanisms associated with the deleterious effects of marijuana use. This chapter provides a neurodevelopmental framework from which recent data on brain structural and functional abnormalities associated with marijuana use is reviewed. Based on the current data, we provide aims for future studies to more clearly delineate the effects of marijuana on the developing brain and to define underlying mechanisms of the potential long-term negative consequences of marijuana use.

International Review of Neurobiology, Volume 129
ISSN 0074-7742
http://dx.doi.org/10.1016/bs.irn.2016.06.004

1. INTRODUCTION

Marijuana is the most commonly used illicit substance in the world and prevalence rates have been increasing over the past decade. Globally, 3–5% of the population above age 15 report current marijuana use, and in the United States 8.4% of the population above age 12 report past month use, with a peak in the 18–25-year age range in which nearly 20% of the population endorse current marijuana use (SAMHSA, 2014; UNODC, 2014). Socially and culturally, use of marijuana has become more widely accepted and viewed as less harmful over the past decade. For example, fewer than 40% of American high school seniors (17–18 years old) reported that they believe it is risky to use marijuana regularly (Johnston, O'Malley, Miech, Bachman, & Schulenberg, 2015), despite the fact that over 4 million Americans experience a marijuana use disorder each year (Center for Behavioral Health Statistics & Quality, 2015). With increased use, changing perceptions of the harmfulness of use, and the movement to decriminalize and even legalize use in numerous locales, it has become crucial to characterize the effects of marijuana on human brain development and function.

Varieties of marijuana (*Cannabis sativa)* contain over 70 identified cannabinoids, of which the primary psychoactive component is Δ^9-tetrahydrocannabinol (THC; ElSohly & Slade, 2005). THC exerts its effects on the endogenous cannabinoid system primarily via cannabinoid-1 (CB1) receptors. CB1 receptors are distributed broadly throughout the brain with particular areas of concentration in prefrontal, cerebellar, temporal, and hippocampal regions (Burns et al., 2007; Glass, Faull, & Dragunow, 1997; cf. Fig. 1B). These brain regions rich in CB1 receptors are instrumental for a wide range of cognitive abilities including executive functioning, reward processing, and memory; thus, the potential effects of THC on brain functioning are equally broad. During acute administration, THC decreases learning and memory (Ranganathan & D'Souza, 2006), psychomotor performance and attention (Ramaekers, Kauert, Theunissen, Toennes, & Moeller, 2009), and reward responsiveness (van Hell et al., 2012), presumably through the alterations of the endocannabinoid system (Rubino et al., 2009). Recent evidence implicates a more complex interaction of THC with both glutamate and γ-aminobutyric acid (GABA) receptors, which may alter more fundamental functions, such as neural oscillatory activity (Raver & Keller, 2014; Rubino & Parolaro, 2016).

Animal models have demonstrated neurotoxic effects of THC (eg, cell shrinkage and damage to DNA structure) particularly in cortical areas with

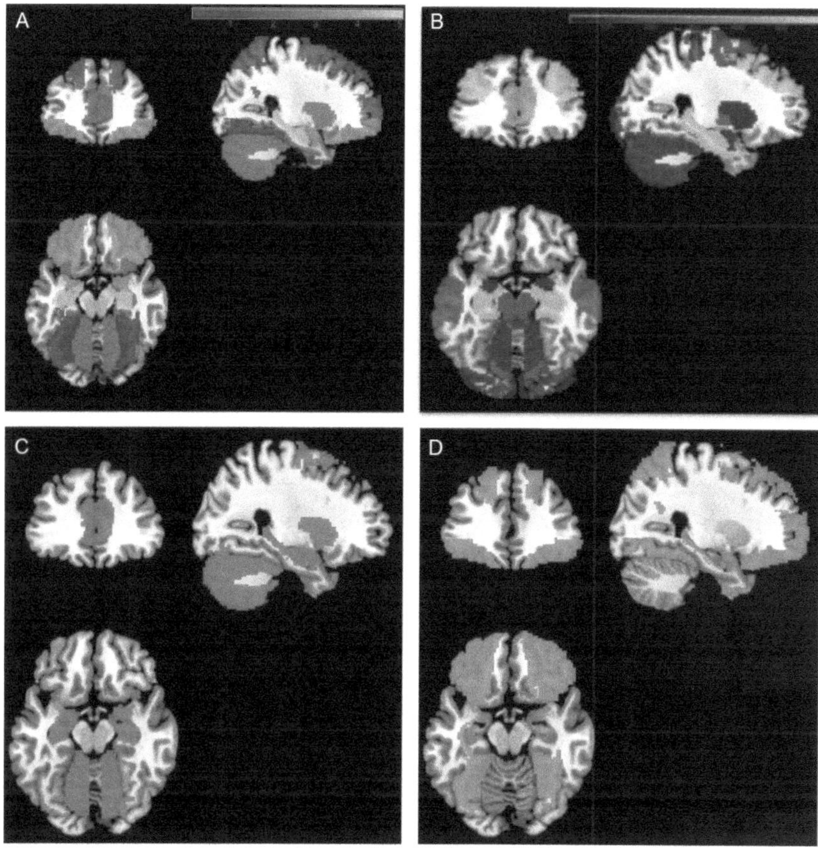

Fig. 1 Weighted color maps. (A) Neuroanatomical alterations in marijuana users (*blue* (*dark gray* in the print version)–green (*light gray* in the print version)), relative to control subjects. (B) Brain map with regional distribution of cannabinoid receptor density [*dark green* (*dark gray* in the print version)–*light green* (*light gray* in the print version); range, 40–1680 density of receptor binding sites, measured via autoradiographic techniques (3)]. Lighter colors indicate evidence from more studies and greater density of receptors. (C) Binary map (*red* (*gray* in the print version)) illustrates overlap between (A) and (B), including regions high in cannabinoid receptors that also show neuroanatomical alterations. (D) Binary map (*violet* (*light gray* in the print version)) illustrates nonoverlap between (A) and (B), including areas that showed neuroanatomic alterations and are low in cannabinoid receptors. *Used with permission from Lorenzetti, V., Solowij, N., & Yücel, M. (2016). The role of cannabinoids on neuroanatomical alterations in cannabis users.* Biological Psychiatry, *79, e17–e31. doi:10.1016/j.biopsych.2015.11.013.*

a high density of CB1 receptors (Chan, Hinds, Impey, & Storm, 1998). THC appears to block synaptic plasticity and neurogenesis, particularly in hippocampal regions, which can have an effect on brain volume (Mato et al., 2004). THC has also been shown to interfere with mesolimbic dopamine pathway functioning (Bossong et al., 2008; Kolb, Gorny, Limebeer, & Parker, 2006). THC activation of CB1 receptors located on GABAergic interneurons in the ventral tegmental area results in increased dopamine release in the nucleus accumbens. This dopamine activity is a common mechanism among drugs of abuse (Cass et al., 2014; Cheer, Wassum, Heien, Phillips, & Wightman, 2004; Gessa, Melis, Muntoni, & Diana, 1998) associated with feelings of reward, reinforcing effects (Kook & Weiss, 1992; Robbin & Everitt, 2002), and drug seeking behaviors (Aarts et al., 2010; Koepp et al., 1998; Urban et al., 2012). By contrast, continued exposure to drugs of abuse is associated with downregulation of dopamine receptors in brain reward systems (Koob & Le Moal, 2001; Koob & Volkow, 2010).

In addition, animal models have demonstrated that exposure to THC during adolescence compared to exposure during adulthood alters maturation of neural networks, particularly in the prefrontal cortex (PFC) and hippocampus (Renard et al., 2016; Rubino & Parolaro, 2016), and results in enduring cognitive deficits (DiNieri & Hurd, 2012; Quinn et al., 2007). For example, exposing rats to THC repeatedly during adolescence resulted in decreased spatial memory performance in adulthood, and this effect seems to be driven by changes in the hippocampus (Rubino et al., 2009). Specifically, rats exposed to THC during adolescence exhibited hippocampal deficits including fewer synaptic connections, less efficient connectivity, and reduced capacity for neuroplasticity (Rubino et al., 2009). In the PFC, Cass et al. (2014) reported that exposure to cannabinoid agonists during early and middle adolescence led to frequency-dependent disinhibition (ie, repeated CB1 receptor stimulation elicits PFC network disinhibition) in adulthood, which was apparently a result of downregulation of GABA transmission. Such modulation of the functioning of the PFC could decrease synaptic plasticity that is essential for the maturation of circuits underlying a broad range of functional domains from decision making to executive functioning (Selemon, 2013). Adolescent exposure to cannabinoid agonists, therefore, can have long lasting effects on the inhibitory and excitatory regulation of the PFC.

Direct downregulation of CB1 receptors may be a key mechanism of marijuana's effects on brain function. Relatively large magnitude adaptations in CB1 receptor functioning are central to the development of tolerance to the behavioral effects of marijuana, but the rate of downregulation and desensitization varies widely by brain region, with PFC exhibiting faster downregulation and basal ganglia exhibiting slower downregulation (Sim-Selley, 2003). Interestingly, in studies utilizing positron emission tomography and FMPEP-d_2, a radioligand for CB1 receptors, the adaptations in CB1 receptors in humans appear largely reversible. Chronic marijuana users exhibited a 20% decrease in cortical CB1 receptors compared to controls at baseline, but after a month of abstinence from marijuana, differences were no longer detectable between users and controls (Hirvonen et al., 2012). In animal models, there is an inverse relationship between CB1 receptor expression in cortical and striatal regions, such that striatal regions with more CB1 receptor expression receive input from cortical regions with less expression, and critically, the expression levels of CB1 receptors in these circuits decrease from adolescence to adulthood (Van Waes, Beverley, Siman, Tseng, & Steiner, 2012; Verdurand et al., 2011). Thus, exogenous influences of THC on these circuits could counteract typical maturational trajectories and yield changes in regions critical for decision making and addiction processes (Volkow & Baler, 2014; Volkow, Koob, & McLellan, 2016).

Studies in humans have demonstrated a number of neurocognitive differences between marijuana users and nonusing controls including impaired verbal learning and memory, attention, psychomotor function, and decision making (Broyd, van Hell, Beale, Yücel, & Solowij, 2016; Volkow, Swanson, et al., 2016). Evidence seems to suggest that some deficits in verbal learning and memory function may recover over time with abstinence (Schreiner & Dunn, 2012); persistent use, however, has been associated with poor long-term neurocognitive performance (Meier et al., 2012) and poorer health outcomes (ie, chronic bronchitis, increased risk of respiratory infections, and vascular conditions such as stroke or infarctions; Volkow, Baler, Compton, & Weiss, 2014). Taken together with animal models showing deficits in brain development when THC is administered during adolescence, it would seem that marijuana use, particularly during this critical developmental period, could negatively affect neurocognitive development. Indeed, individuals who begin using marijuana during adolescence exhibit lower IQs and seem to have less crystallized intelligence (ie, acquired knowledge through skills and experience; Jackson et al., 2016). At the same time, the direct effect of marijuana use on neurocognitive deteriorations during adolescence has not been shown to be significantly related to frequency of use, and may be attributable to genetic or familial factors that contribute to risk for both marijuana use initiation and low intellectual achievement (Jackson et al., 2016). Therefore, characterizing changes in brain structure and function related to marijuana use may help differentiate risk factors from consequences of marijuana use. Careful study design is necessary to overcome some of the inherent challenges in illustrating specific effects of marijuana, as marijuana use often cooccurs with alcohol and nicotine consumption, and heritable factors (eg, genetics and personality traits) likely contribute to brain differences independent of marijuana use (Hurd, Michaelides, Miller, & Jutras-Aswad, 2014).

In the current chapter, we will (1) describe a neurodevelopmental framework for understanding the effects of marijuana use on brain structure and function, (2) summarize the robust results and discuss recent findings from neuroimaging studies of the effects of marijuana use on brain structure and function, and (3) highlight remaining questions and areas of ongoing evaluation in understanding the effects of marijuana use on the human brain.

2. NEURODEVELOPMENTAL FRAMEWORK FOR UNDERSTANDING THE EFFECTS OF MARIJUANA ON BRAIN STRUCTURE AND FUNCTION

The human brain continues to mature throughout adolescence, a time during which dramatic changes occur in neurochemistry and anatomy including both cortical and hormonal alterations (Giedd et al., 1999; Gogtay et al., 2004; Luciana, 2013; Raznahan et al., 2011). Gray matter (GM) decreases following an inverted *U*-shaped developmental progression—peaking in childhood and decreasing through the early 20s (Giedd et al., 1999, 2009). The measures of GM (cortical thickness (CT), surface area (SA), and their product, cortical volume) follow different developmental trajectories with CT peaking between 2 and 4 years of age and then steadily declining through adulthood, while SA increases up to roughly age 12 before leveling off through age 30 (Amlien et al., 2014; Walhovd, Fjell, Giedd, Dale, & Brown, 2016). The trajectories of CT and SA yield the cortical GM volumes that decrease from around ages 10–12 through adulthood. Normally, age-related decreases in GM localized to the prefrontal and temporal cortices (Giedd et al., 1999; Gogtay et al., 2004) and in subcortical structures, including the striatum and thalamus (Sowell, Thompson, Holmes, Jernigan, & Toga, 1999; Toga, Thompson, & Sowell, 2006), are attributed to pruning of excessive neurons and to cortical myelination (Huttenlocher & Dabholkar, 1997; Shaw et al., 2008).

White matter (WM) volume increases linearly during adolescence through young adulthood (Giedd et al., 1999, 2009), yielding relatively stable total brain volumes after puberty. WM maturation is associated with greater structural connectivity between brain regions and, consequently, more efficient communication between frontal and subcortical regions (Sowell et al., 1999; Toga et al., 2006). In addition to increasing volume of WM, the quality of the microstructure continues to mature to more efficient and well-connected networks. Common measures from diffusion tensor imaging (DTI) used to infer WM microstructure include fractional anisotropy (FA), or directionally restricted diffusion of water, radial diffusivity (RD), or the perpendicular diffusion of water, and mean diffusivity (MD), or the overall magnitude of diffusion. Increasing FA is associated with more efficient and mature WM, while higher RD and MD are associated with less efficient WM. FA increases throughout adolescence and young adulthood with a relatively stable peak between 20 and 40 years, while RD and MD tend to reflect the opposite trends with decreases through adolescence and young adulthood with a relatively stable minimum between 18 and 40 years of age (Bava et al., 2010; Lebel et al., 2012). These general developmental trajectories form the basis for understanding and interpreting potential changes associated with marijuana use.

The peak incidence of marijuana use occurs in later adolescence and early adulthood, so, it is critical to approach questions of marijuana effects on brain structure and function from a developmental perspective. Casey, Oliveri, and Insel (2014) presented a neurodevelopmental framework that is useful for conceptualizing critical questions of potential alterations to development by outside factors, such as drugs of abuse. The first concept is developmental trajectories, which is largely described by the extant literature on adolescent brain development. Starting from these well-established developmental trajectories, summarized earlier, allows us to describe alterations in terms of delays, deviations, or regressions from normal trajectories.

The second concept is sensitive periods, or windows of development in which the brain may be uniquely malleable and perhaps susceptible to influences that could alter its trajectory (Casey et al., 2014). The changes occurring in the adolescent brain, characterized by plasticity and maturational changes, represent both opportunities and vulnerabilities that make this developmental period critical (Dahl, 2004; Fuhrmann, Knoll, & Blakemore, 2015; Luciana, 2013). This concept is relevant to the goal of identifying developmentally defined epochs of exposure to marijuana that yield stronger and perhaps more deleterious effects on developmental trajectories.

The third concept is dynamic interaction of systems (Casey et al., 2014). Comprehending the developmental cascades at play in determining the effects of marijuana use on brain structure and function requires sophisticated models of complex interactions. Making attempts to characterize the interaction of multiple brain systems maturing at different rates over adolescence and early adulthood will be critical for understanding how environmental events (eg, onset of marijuana use) may modulate the function or development of these systems. Furthermore, capturing synergism between genetics, behavioral traits, and experience is a vital and complex process. As we summarize results from imaging studies of the effects of marijuana use on the brain in humans, we will frequently refer to these concepts to help guide interpretations and to delineate questions and areas for future investigations.

3. STRUCTURAL CHANGES ASSOCIATED WITH MARIJUANA USE

3.1 Gray Matter

Neuroanatomic differences in GM between marijuana users and healthy controls have been reported in several specific regions, but there is very little evidence of global differences in intracranial volume or total GM volume (Lorenzetti, Solowij, Fornito, Ian Lubman, & Yucel, 2014). Many studies have reported smaller volumes in regions rich in CB1 receptors in marijuana users, and while several studies have summarized large portions of this literature (Batalla et al., 2013; Bhattacharyya, Atakan, Martin-Santos, Crippa, & McGuire, 2012; Lorenzetti et al., 2014; Lorenzetti, Solowij, & Yücel, 2016; Martín-Santos et al., 2010), we will summarize the most robust findings here while also highlighting recent reports (ie, since 2010; Table 1 and Fig. 1).

Smaller hippocampal volumes in marijuana users relative to healthy controls have been one of the most consistently reported findings (Ashtari et al., 2011; Demirakca et al., 2011; Lorenzetti et al., 2015; Matochik, Eldreth, Cadet, & Bolla, 2005; Schacht, Hutchison, & Filbey, 2012; Yucel et al., 2008). These studies reported cross-sectional comparisons of marijuana users and nonusing controls with varying levels of marijuana use history, and many studies examining the effect of dosage or lifetime exposure show an inverse relationship between use and hippocampal volume, with more

Table 1 Recent Studies (2010–2015) Comparing Morphometric Brain Measures with Marijuana Users and Nonusers

Authors	Key Findings	Groups	*n*	Age Range Mean (SD) [Range]	Sex % Male
Ashtari et al. (2011)	MJ < CON volume in right and left hippocampus; In MJ smaller hippocampus volume = more use	MJ *abstinent 30 + days—mean 6 months*	14	19.3 (0.8) [18–20]	100%
		CON	14	18.5 (1.4) [18–20]	100%
Battistella et al. (2014)	RMJ < OMJ volume in the medial temporal cortex, temporal pole, parahippocampal gyrus, insula, and orbitofrontal cortex; Lower age of onset = smaller volumes RMJ > OMJ volume in cerebellum	OMJ	22	25 (2.8)[a] [19–29]	100%
		RMJ	23	23 (2.2) [20–28]	100%
Churchwell et al. (2010)	MJ < CON volume in right medial orbital PFC; Lower age of onset = smaller volumes	MJ	18	17.7 (0.9) [16–19]	89%
		CON	18	17.2 (0.8) [16–19]	67%
Cousijn et al. (2012)	MJ > CON volume in anterior cerebellum; Within MJ higher use = smaller volume in amygdala and hippocampus	MJ	33	21.3 (2.4) [18–25]	64%
		CON	42	21.9 (2.4) [18–25]	62%
Demirakca et al. (2011)	MJ < CON volume in right hippocampus; Within MJ higher THC in THC/CBD ratio = smaller volume	MJ	11	*NR* [19–25][b]	100%
		CON	13	*NR* [19–25][b]	100%
Filbey et al. (2014)	MJ = MJ only < CON volume in right middle OFC, and left superior OFC	MJ	48	28.3 (8.3) [*NR*]	69%
		MJ only *No alcohol use*	27	28.1 (8.9) [*NR*]	63%
		CON	62	30.0 (7.4) [*NR*]	63%

Continued

Table 1 Recent Studies (2010–2015) Comparing Morphometric Brain Measures with Marijuana Users and Nonusers—cont'd

Authors	Key Findings	Groups	*n*	Age Range Mean (SD) [Range]	Sex % Male
Filbey et al. (2015)	MJ early *with more use* > MJ late *with more use* thickness in anterior dorsolateral frontal cortex (moderator effect)	MJ early *onset < age 16*	20	32.5 (8.01) [21–50]	55%
		MJ late *onset > age 16*	22	30.3 (7.19) [21–47]	73%
Gilman et al. (2014)	MJ > CON GM density in left nucleus accumbens, hypothalamus, sublenticular extended amygdala, and left amygdala; Significant shape differences in left nucleus accumbens and right amygdala	MJ	20	21.3 (1.9) [18–25]	45%
		CON	20	20.7 (1.9) [18–25]	45%
Jacobus et al. (2015)	MJ + ALC > CON thickness across frontal and parietal regions; MJ > CON (*controlling for alcohol*) thickness in left temporal and right entorhinal cortices	MJ + ALC	30	Baseline: 18.2 (0.8) [16–19] Year 1.5: 19.6 (0.8) Year 3: 21.2 (0.7)	63%
		CON	38	Baseline: 17.7 (0.9) [16–19] Year 1.5: 19.1 (0.9) Year 3: 20.8 (1.0)	76%
Lopez-Larson et al. (2011)	MJ < CON thickness in right caudal middle frontal, bilateral insula, and bilateral superior frontal regions MJ > CON thickness in the bilateral lingual, right superior temporal, right inferior parietal and left paracentral regions Within MJ lower age of onset = thicker right superior frontal gyrus	MJ	18	17.8 (1.0) [16–19]	94.4%
		CON	18	17.3 (0.8) [16–19]	66.6%

Lorenzetti et al. (2015)	MJ < CON volume in hippocampus and amygdala	MJ	15	40 (9) [*NR*]	100%
		CON	15	36 (10) [*NR*]	100%
Medina et al. (2010)	MJ > CON volume in inferior posterior vermis (cerebellum)	MJ	16	18.11 (0.74) [16–18]	75%
		CON	16	18.01 (0.97) [16–18]	63%
Schacht et al. (2012)	MJ < CON volume in hippocampus and left amygdala MJ < CON CB1 receptor genetic variation (rs2023239 G allele) = lower volume hippocampus (group × time interaction)	MJ full	94	24.2 (7.4) [*NR*]	34%
		MJ matched	37	27.8 (8.7) [*NR*]	37%
		CON	37	27.3 (7.9) [*NR*]	37%
Weiland et al. (2015)	No volume or shape differences in subcortical structures examined (nucleus accumbens, amygdala, hippocampus, and cerebellum)	Adult MJ	29	27.4 (7.1) [19–53]	55%
		Adult CON	29	27.5 (6.8) [18–53]	55%
		Adol MJ	50	16.7 (1.1) [14–18]	82%
		Adol CON	50	16.8 (1.0) [14–18]	72%
Yip et al. (2014)	MJ < CON volume in putamen Within MJ smaller putamen volume = higher probability of relapse	MJ *dependent*	20	26.7 (2.2) [*NR*]	100%
		CON	20	29.2 (2.3) [*NR*]	100%

Notes: *ALC*, alcohol use group; *CON*, control group; *MJ*, marijuana use group; *MJ + ALC*, marijuana and alcohol use group; *NR*, not reported; *OMJ*, occasional marijuana use group; *RMJ*, regular marijuana use group.
[a]Median (SD).
[b]No means provided but groups were reported as equal.

use resulting in smaller volumes (Ashtari et al., 2011; Matochik et al., 2005; Yucel et al., 2008). In a sample that did not exhibit group differences between marijuana users and controls, higher lifetime marijuana use within the marijuana-using group was associated with smaller hippocampal volumes (Cousijn et al., 2012). Thus, dose and duration appear critical for effects of marijuana on hippocampal volume.

Other factors may also contribute to smaller hippocampal volumes in marijuana users. For example, in a small sample of young adults, higher levels of THC relative to cannabidiol (CBD) in a hair sample, reflecting use over the past 4–5 months, was associated with smaller hippocampal volumes (Demirakca et al., 2011). Furthermore, an examination of genetic variants of a CB1 receptor gene (ie, rs2023239) provided evidence that genes may interact with marijuana use, as carriers of the G allele who used marijuana exhibited smaller hippocampal volumes compared with healthy controls carrying the G allele, as well as compared with marijuana-using carriers of the A allele (Schacht et al., 2012). Identifying a genetic component that may interact with marijuana use is an important step in differentiating risk factors for marijuana use from outcomes of THC toxicity following marijuana use.

In addition to effects on hippocampal volume, several studies have reported consequences of marijuana use on the amygdala and striatum, including increased GM density (likely reflecting denser dendritic branching; Gilman et al., 2014; Matochik et al., 2005), and decreased volumes (Lorenzetti et al., 2015; Schacht et al., 2012; Yip et al., 2014). In other structures, associations between marijuana use and brain volumes are less well delineated. For example, in marijuana users compared to controls, one study reported a slight increase in accumbens volume (Gilman et al., 2014), another reported greater GM density in the left nucleus accumbens extending to subcallosal cortex, hypothalamus, and amygdala (Gilman et al., 2014), and marijuana use has also been associated with smaller and thinner insular cortex (Battistella et al., 2014; Lopez-Larson et al., 2011).

The cerebellum, noted as a key target of marijuana exposure in imaging studies, is a region rich in CB1 receptors. Two studies that included adolescents and young adults reported larger cerebellar volumes among marijuana users compared to controls (Cousijn et al., 2012; Medina, Nagel, & Tapert, 2010), while a study in a much older sample with a longer history of marijuana use reported smaller cerebellar volumes compared to controls (Solowij et al., 2011). Additionally, in a large study that recruited a sample of adult marijuana users and controls and a sample of adolescent marijuana users and controls, no significant differences in volume were found in subcortical structures (eg, amygdala, hippocampus, and cerebellum) in either sample (Weiland et al., 2015). Weiland et al. (2015) highlight that their marijuana users and controls were matched on alcohol use severity using the Alcohol Use Disorders Identification Test (AUDIT); however, characterizing marijuana use groups based on the past 2 months (for adults) and past 3 months (for adolescents) of use limited their ability to examine effects of cumulative lifetime use or age of onset.

The morphometry of PFC is also affected by marijuana use (Fig. 1). Specifically, marijuana use has been associated with smaller volumes in the orbitofrontal cortex (OFC; Battistella et al., 2014; Churchwell, Lopez-Larson, & Yurgelun-Todd, 2010; Filbey et al., 2014) and with thinner cortices in caudal middle frontal regions (Lopez-Larson et al., 2011). Interestingly, age of onset was negatively correlated with thickness in two studies (Filbey, McQueeny, DeWitt, & Mishra, 2015; Lopez-Larson et al., 2011). In both, earlier onset of marijuana use (ie, before age 16) was associated with thicker PFC. Lopez-Larson et al. (2011) examined participants while they were still adolescents (ie, 16–19 years old) and reported a negative correlation between age of onset of regular marijuana use and the superior frontal gyrus, whereas Filbey et al. (2015) collected data on older participants (ie, 21–50 years old) and reported that those who initiated marijuana use before age 16 exhibited thicker anterior dorsolateral PFC. Taken together, these findings demonstrate that early marijuana use onset interacts with cortical development during adolescence, likely leading to the disruption of typical development (eg, pruning and plasticity).

As mentioned, the majority of currently published data on the effects of marijuana use on GM is cross-sectional; very few studies have examined changes over time using longitudinal methods. One study utilizing a single MRI acquisition at age 12 to predict substance use outcomes, at age 16 reported that smaller OFC (but not amygdala, hippocampus, or anterior cingulate cortex) volumes were associated with a greater probability of initiation of marijuana use by age 16 (Cheetham et al., 2012). The authors controlled for other substance use and also examined whether smaller OFC volumes predicted the onset of other substance use, and reported that OFC volumes were uniquely associated with the onset of marijuana use. Thus, regional volume in the OFC appears to be specifically related to THC use, and could be a potential risk marker for initiating and maintaining marijuana use.

Some of the only studies to date that have utilized longitudinal MRI data to examine the effects of marijuana use have come out of our group (Tapert and colleagues). For example, we recently examined CT over 3 years of late adolescence (18–21 years old) in a sample of heavy marijuana and alcohol users compared to controls (Jacobus et al., 2015). Substance users exhibited thicker cortices in all four lobes of the brain that persisted over the 3-year period, which might reflect a reduction in expected developmental pruning. Thickness measures trended downward in both groups, as expected, but the substance-using sample exhibited a shallower decline compared to controls (eg, in the paracentral lobule). Furthermore, when controlling for alcohol use, lifetime marijuana use was positively associated with CT while age of onset of marijuana use was negatively associated with CT in the temporal lobe, indicating that some of the observed differences were likely specific to marijuana use. Another recent study, examining 16–18-year-old participants over 18 months described similar attenuation of CT declines (ie, shallower slope of change) in marijuana users compared to controls (Epstein & Kumra, 2015a). These longitudinal data largely support reports from cross-sectional studies, and underscore the concept that changes in cortical morphometry are dynamic and influenced by preexisting vulnerabilities as well as by different levels of neurotoxicity or attenuated neuroplasticity related to dose, duration, and age of onset of marijuana use.

3.2 White Matter

A majority of studies examining WM integrity in cross-sectional samples of adolescent and adult marijuana users have reported decreased FA and increased MD and RD indicating less efficient or less mature WM microstructure in users compared to controls in widely dispersed brain regions (Table 2). For example, central WM regions such as the genu, rostrum, and splenium of the corpus callosum (Arnone et al., 2008; Gruber, Dahlgren, Sagar, Gönenç, & Lukas, 2014; Gruber, Silveri, Dahlgren, & Yurgelun-Todd, 2011), as well as the superior longitudinal fasciculus and arcuate fasciculus (Ashtari, Cervellione, Cottone, Ardekani, & Kumra, 2009; Bava et al., 2009; Thatcher, Pajtek, Chung, Terwilliger, & Clark, 2010) show higher FA in controls compared to marijuana users. Some studies report increased FA (ie, purportedly more efficient or mature WM) among users in regions such as the forceps minor (Filbey et al., 2014) and the internal capsule and superior longitudinal fasciculus (Bava et al., 2009), though such results are tentative since DTI findings can be affected by important covariates such as age of onset of marijuana use (Gruber et al., 2014, 2011) and sex (Thatcher et al., 2010).

Table 2 Recent Studies (2009–2015) Comparing White Matter Integrity Measures Between Marijuana Users and Nonusers

Authors	Key Findings	Groups	*n*	Age Range Mean (SD) [Range]	Sex % Male
Ashtari et al. (2009)	MJ < CON FA in arcuate fasciculus MJ < CON RD in arcuate fasciculus	MJ *abstinent 30+ days*	14	19.3 (0.8) [18–21]	100%
		CON	14	18.5 (1.4) [17–21]	100%
Bava et al. (2009)	MJ + ALC < CON FA in left superior longitudinal fasciculus, left postcentral gyrus, bilateral crus cerebri, and inferior frontal and temporal tracts MJ + ALC > CON FA in right occipital, internal capsule, and superior longitudinal fasciculus	MJ + ALC	36	17.9 (0.9) [16–19]	72%
		CON	36	17.8 (0.8) [16–19]	72%
Bava et al. (2013)	MJ + ALC < CON FA in right splenium, right prefrontal thalamic fibers, and right corona radiate at baseline and 18 months MJ + ALC > CON MD & RD in superior longitudinal fasciculus, right posterior thalamic radiations, right prefrontal thalamic fibers, right superior temporal gyrus, right inferior longitudinal fasciculus, and left posterior corona radiate at baseline and 18 months	MJ + ALC	41	Time 1: 18.4 (1.2) [16–21] Time 2: 19.8 (1.1) [17–22]	73%
		CON	51	Time 1: 17.9 (1.1) [16–21] Time 2: 19.3 (1.1) [17–22]	63%

Continued

Table 2 Recent Studies (2009–2015) Comparing White Matter Integrity Measures Between Marijuana Users and Nonusers—cont'd

Authors	Key Findings	Groups	*n*	Age Range Mean (SD) [Range]	Sex % Male
Becker et al. (2015)	MJ > CON FA in genu, forceps minor; MJ < CON growth in FA in superior longitudinal fasciculus, left superior frontal gyrus, left corticospinal tract, and right anterior thalamic radiation Within MJ higher use = reduced longitudinal growth in FA	MJ	23	Time 1: 19.5 (0.7) [18–20] Time 2 + 2.2 (0.5)	70%
		CON	23	Time 1: 19.2 (2.3) [15–23] Time 2: +2.2 (0.5) years	70%
Epstein and Kumra (2015b)[a]	MJ < CON FA in inferior longitudinal fasciculus over 18 months More use over 18 months = lower FA	MJ	19	Baseline: 16.6 (1.5) Year 1.5: +1.5 years	58%
		CON	29	Baseline: 16.5 (2.2) Year 1.5: +1.5 years	45%
Filbey et al. (2014)	MJ > CON FA in forceps minor MJ < CON RD in forceps minor	MJ	48	28.3 (8.3) [*NR*]	69%
		MJ exc *marijuana use only*	27	28.1 (8.9) [*NR*]	63%
		CON	62	30.0 (7.4) [*NR*]	63%
Gruber et al. (2014)	MJ < CON FA in genu and left internal capsule MJ < CON MD in genu Within MJ earlier age onset = lower FA	MJ	25	23.1 (3.5) [*NR*]	72.0%
		CON	18	23.2 (5.9) [*NR*]	38.9%

Gruber et al. (2011)	MJ < CON FA in left frontal regions Within MJ earlier age onset = lower FA	MJ	15	25 (8.7) [*NR*]	93.3%
		CON	15	25.2 (8.4)	93.3%
Jacobus, McQueeny, et al. (2009)	MJ + ALC < CON FA in corona radiate and superior longitudinal fasciculus ALC < CON FA in corona radiata, inferior longitudinal fasciculus, inferior fronto-occipital fasciculus, cerebellar peduncle, and superior longitudinal fasciculus MJ + ALC > ALC FA in corona radiata, inferior fronto-occipital fasciculus, cerebellar peduncle, and superior longitudinal fasciculus	MJ + ALC	14	18.2 (0.7) [16–19]	79%
		ALC	14	18.1 (0.7) [16–19]	86%
		CON	14	17.3 (0.8) [16–19]	86%
Jacobus, Thayer, et al. (2013)	Within MJ + ALC lower FA in fornix and superior corona radiata at time 1 = higher substance use and risk taking at time 2	MJ + ALC	47	Time 1: 18.0 (0.9) [16–19] Time 2: 19.5 (0.9)	59%
		CON	49	Time 1: 17.6 (0.8) [16–19] Time 2: 19.0 (0.9)	73%
Jacobus, Squeglia, Infante, et al. (2013)	MJ decreased FA from time 1 to time 2 (12 clusters) MJ decreased and ALC increased FA from time 1 to time 2 (6 clusters)	MJ initiators	8	Time 1: 18.2 (0.7) [17–19] Time 2: 21.2 (*NR*) [20–22]	*NR*
		ALC initiators	8	Time 1: 17.5 (0.8) [17–19] Time 2: 20.6 (*NR*) [20–23]	*NR*

Continued

Table 2 Recent Studies (2009–2015) Comparing White Matter Integrity Measures Between Marijuana Users and Nonusers—cont'd

Authors	Key Findings	Groups	*n*	Age Range Mean (SD) [Range]	Sex % Male
Jacobus, Squeglia, Bava, et al. (2013)	MJ + ALC = ALC < CON FA in 14 clusters ALC < MJ + ALC < CON FA in uncinate fasciculus MJ + ALC = MJ = decrease FA from baseline to year 3 in 12 clusters	MJ + ALC	21	Baseline: 17.9 (*NR*) [16–19] Year 1.5: 19.4 (*NR*) [17–20] Year 3: 20.9 (*NR*) [19–21]	62%
		ALC	17	Baseline: 17.9 (*NR*) [16–19] Year 1.5: 19.3 (*NR*) [17–20] Year 3: 20.9 (*NR*) [19–22]	64%
		CON	16	Baseline: 17.9 (*NR*) [16–19] Year 1.5: 19.4 (*NR*) [17–20] Year 3: 20.9 (*NR*) [19–22]	50%
Zalesky et al. (2012)	MJ < CON WM connectivity in the right fimbria of the hippocampus (fornix), splenium of the corpus callosum, and commissural fibers Within MJ lower age of onset = higher RD	MJ	59	33.4 (10.9) [*NR*]	47%
		CON	33	31.5 (12.0) [*NR*]	42%

Notes: *ALC*, alcohol use group; *CON*, control group; *FA*, fractional anisotropy; *MJ*, marijuana use group; *MJ + ALC*, marijuana and alcohol use group; *NR*, not reported; *RD*, radial diffusivity; *MD*, mean diffusivity; *WM*, white matter.

[a]An early-onset schizophrenia group was reported in this study, but is not summarized here.

In order to elucidate some of complexities from the many cross-sectional studies on marijuana's effects on WM, our lab reported on a series of longitudinal studies of late adolescence. We found that over an 18-month follow-up period of continued use, heavy marijuana and alcohol use resulted in systematically lower FA and higher MD, specifically in the superior longitudinal fasciculus, right posterior thalamic radiations, right prefrontal thalamic fibers, right superior temporal gyrus, right inferior longitudinal fasciculus, and left posterior corona radiata (Bava, Jacobus, Thayer, & Tapert, 2013). Marijuana use did not independently predict these effects, but drinking predicted decreased FA and increased MD over the follow-up period. Another recent study reported that 16–18-year-old marijuana users exhibited decreasing FA values in the inferior longitudinal fasciculus over 18 months compared to healthy controls (Epstein & Kumra, 2015b).

In a separate longitudinal study including three groups of adolescents (heavy drinkers, heavy drinkers and heavy marijuana users, and controls) examined over 3 years (ie, 18–21), we found that controls exhibited greater FA than both user groups across the majority of regions examined and that both user groups exhibited lower FA values at each time point over the 3 years (Jacobus, Squeglia, Bava, & Tapert, 2013). The substance-using groups differed in only one region, the right uncinate fasciculus, where the heavy drinking and marijuana-using group exhibited higher FA than the heavy drinking only group. We further examined a group of adolescents who reported little substance use at baseline (16–18 years old), but then initiated either alcohol or marijuana by the 3-year follow-up assessment (19–22 years old) to try to parse out premorbid WM differences from those related to substance use (Jacobus, Squeglia, Infante, Bava, & Tapert, 2013). In this small study ($n=8$ alcohol initiators and $n=8$ alcohol and marijuana initiators), we found decreasing FA in the alcohol and marijuana group, but not in the alcohol-only group across 20 different brain regions. This study, while preliminary, represents one of the only studies to date that has examined WM microstructure prior to and after the initiation of alcohol and marijuana use in adolescents and highlights a number of regions (ie, splenium of the corpus callosum, forceps minor, fronto-occipital fasciculus, superior corona radiata, posterior corona radiata, corticospinal tract, internal capsule, uncinated fasciculus, and superior longitudinal fasciculus) of interest for future studies.

Another longitudinal examination of WM over 2 years of late adolescence/early adulthood (ie, 19–21 years old) conducted by Becker, Collins, Lim, Muetzel, and Luciana (2015) compared heavy marijuana users who concurrently used alcohol, with controls who had no marijuana and limited alcohol use (Becker et al., 2015). Their group reported higher FA and lower RD in the controls compared to substance users over 2 years in the superior longitudinal fasciculus and corticospinal tract. Marijuana users also exhibited higher FA, particularly in the right genu of the corpus callosum. Interestingly, the authors found that higher levels of marijuana use reported in the past 12 months at follow-up was negatively associated with FA in the superior longitudinal fasciculus and corticospinal tract. While the marijuana-using group also reported significantly more alcohol use than the control group, alcohol use was unrelated to the observed FA changes over the 2 years. These results are consistent with our smaller study examining the onset of marijuana and alcohol use, in that marijuana and alcohol, but not alcohol alone, were associated with greater WM deficits.

The WM alterations associated with marijuana use are likely attributable to effects on pruning and myelination processes occurring during adolescence and early adulthood (Lebel et al., 2012) and could underlie functional alterations later in life. For example, Filbey et al. (2014) examined a sample of adult marijuana users and found they exhibited smaller OFC volumes, but greater functional connectivity in the OFC. Another group reported the same increased OFC functional connectivity in a sample of 14–20 years old adolescent and young adult marijuana users (Lopez-Larson, Rogowska, & Yurgelun-Todd, 2015). Similar results have been reported in resting state data (Orr et al., 2013) and in functional connectivity underlying cognitive control tasks (Harding et al., 2012). The authors postulate that the increased functional connectivity coupled with decreased volume and structural connectivity in WM tracts (ie, decreased FA), may indicate a compensatory mechanism or "neural scaffolding" effect, wherein neurodevelopmental trajectories are modulated by exposure to marijuana and result in long-term functional alterations (Filbey et al., 2014). To explore the functional consequences of structural differences related to marijuana use further, we will briefly review findings related to functional brain imaging studies.

4. FUNCTIONAL MRI OBSERVATIONS IN MARIJUANA USE

Several recent reviews have summarized the consequences of marijuana use on neurocognitive functioning in adolescence (Jackson et al., 2016) and adulthood (Auer, Vittinghoff, Yaffe, et al., 2016; Broyd et al.,

2016), and have highlighted deficits in verbal memory, processing speed, and executive functioning (Volkow, Swanson, et al., 2016). Presumably functional MRI studies reflect the brain changes underlying the long-term neurocognitive deficits; however, the connection between structural brain changes and functional manifestations has not been clearly defined. For example, our lab has described fMRI findings from spatial working memory (Padula, Schweinsburg, & Tapert, 2007; Schweinsburg et al., 2008, 2005; Schweinsburg, Schweinsburg, Medina, et al., 2010), verbal encoding (Schweinsburg, McQueeny, Nagel, Eyler, & Tapert, 2010), and inhibitory control tasks (Tapert et al., 2007), and in each case marijuana users and controls demonstrated similar task performance, but the underlying brain activation patterns differed significantly. In our studies, marijuana users' relative to controls' brain function was characterized by increased activation in parietal, superior temporal, hippocampal, and posterior cingulate regions during working memory demands, and increased parietal and frontal activation during response inhibition.

Other studies in young adults have corroborated the differential activation depicted in our adolescent samples, including a study that reported hypoactivity in frontal and temporal cortices, and relative hyperactivity in the parahippocampal region during a learning task (Nestor, Roberts, Garavan, & Hester, 2008), and a study that reported greater activation in marijuana users compared to controls in frontal and temporal regions during a visuospatial working memory task (Smith, Longo, Fried, Hogan, & Cameron, 2010). In each of these cases, marijuana users and controls performed similarly on the tasks, but exhibited differential brain activation reflecting potential compensatory responses by the marijuana-using groups (Filbey et al., 2015; Schweinsburg, McQueeny, et al., 2010).

Age of onset and amount of marijuana consumed appear to modulate fMRI results. Earlier onset and more intense marijuana use during adolescence was linked to less brain activation (ie, BOLD response), and users who began using marijuana in late adolescence showed notably higher brain activation compared to earlier onset users (Jacobus, Bava, Cohen-Zion, Mahmood, & Tapert, 2009). A recent study examining performance on a Stroop task in adults showed that marijuana users performed poorly on the task compared to controls, and also exhibited a different pattern of activation in the cingulate compared to controls (Sagar et al., 2015). Specifically, the subset of marijuana smokers with an onset of regular use prior to age 16 exhibited significant activation in the anterior cingulate, which was not evident in the late onset marijuana users or controls (Sagar et al.,

2015). Thus, the weakened capacity of marijuana users to rely on brain regions typically required for task execution (eg, executive functioning and working memory) appears to result in the recruitment of additional brain regions associated with attentional or verbal processing that are not typically utilized.

Marijuana use appears to affect the mesolimbic dopamine system, a target of many, if not all other drugs of abuse (Filbey & DeWitt, 2012). Tasks requiring brain reward systems revealed a similar constellation of results; namely, that marijuana users and controls did not differ in their performance of the tasks, but exhibited differential activation of reward pathways, including increased activation of regions of the basal ganglia (ie, caudate, putamen, and nucleus accumbens) and the insula (Hester, Nestor, & Garavan, 2009; van Hell et al., 2010) during reward anticipation. Additionally, marijuana users exhibited decreased activation in the insula, anterior cingulate, and putamen during loss trials in a monetary incentive delay task (Nestor, Hester, & Garavan, 2010; Wesley, Hanlon, & Porrino, 2011). Thus, marijuana users may be more sensitive to rewards and less sensitive to negative feedback or losses.

In summary, functional MRI studies reveal relatively intact performance that is accomplished with differential activation patterns in marijuana users compared to controls. The data support a hypothesis of expanding neural recruitment that entails compensatory activation in brain regions not typically utilized to accomplish the task. Future studies with more difficult neurocognitive tasks and over a larger range of ages may provide additional evidence and clarify underlying functional changes resulting from marijuana use.

5. REMAINING QUESTIONS AND FUTURE DIRECTIONS

The literature on brain structure and function is beginning to elucidate the specific and primarily detrimental effects of marijuana use, particularly when initiated while the brain is still maturing during early to mid-adolescence. Data indicates that adolescence is indeed a sensitive period in development in which marijuana use can result in long-term negative effects. Additional research is needed to clarify the developmental trajectories of neurobiological systems including the endocannabinoid system and related neuronal systems, and to more clearly characterize the effects of marijuana use on these systems. Complex interactions between the development of the endocannabinoid system with other factors including genetics

(Schacht et al., 2012), age of use onset (Gruber et al., 2014), and behavioral traits (Wesley et al., 2011) will be crucial to untangle in future studies (Hurd et al., 2014). In order to obtain data capable of addressing some of these issues, a number of methodological and conceptual advancements must also be considered in the coming years.

One such advancement is a clearer depiction of the mechanisms of action of marijuana's effects on the developing brain. Much of the neurotoxic effects of marijuana are associated with THC acting on CB1 receptors, which in turn affects a number of other neurotransmitter systems and neurodevelopmental processes (eg, synaptic plasticity and neurogenesis in the hippocampus; Lubman, Cheetham, & Yücel, 2015). THC is only one of more than 70 cannabinoids in marijuana and not all of these cannabinoids have neurotoxic effects. In fact CBD may even counteract some of the negative effects of THC (Bhattacharyya et al., 2010; Demirakca et al., 2011). Additional studies are needed to parse out the potentially countervailing effects of different cannabinoids.

In order to better understand the complex effects of marijuana, researchers also need to improve assessment techniques. The majority of marijuana use data come from self-report and are quantified with crude measures of "days of use," "number of joints," or "grams" consumed. While it is inherently difficult to quantify an unregulated substance, it is clear that potency of marijuana has been steadily increasing and different methods of administration inevitably lead to different active doses (ElSohly et al., 2016). Therefore, developing better and more standardized assessment techniques is essential to addressing the complexities of THC doses and potency (Lorenzetti et al., 2016). It is possible, for example, to utilize hair samples that will provide an index of use over 3–5 months and also provide a basic ratio of THC and CBD (Demirakca et al., 2011). As toxicology tests of urine and other bodily fluids continue to improve (Hartman et al., 2015, 2016), researchers will need to update current methods and incorporate additional techniques to address some of these fundamental questions of pharmacokinetics and pharmacodynamics of marijuana.

Lastly, researchers must collect longitudinal data that can disentangle precursors of risk from consequences of marijuana use. Nearly, all of the existing imaging literature on the effects of marijuana on neurodevelopment is cross-sectional in nature and cannot address questions of cause and effect. Approaching these questions from a neurodevelopmental perspective requires understanding of (1) typical trajectories, (2) sensitive periods, and (3) complex interactions at multiple levels (Casey et al., 2014). None of these aims can be sufficiently addressed solely with cross-sectional data. Fortunately, funding organizations have recently prioritized large scale, longitudinal studies, which will provide data to address some of the remaining questions. For example, in the United States, the National Institutes of Health funded the National Consortium on Alcohol and Neuro-Development in Adolescence (http://www.ncanda.org) to examine the effects of alcohol and other drugs on neurodevelopmental trajectories in a large sample ($n=831$) of adolescents including annual neuroimaging and neurocognitive assessments (Brown et al., 2015; Pfefferbaum et al., 2015); the European Union has funded the IMAGEN project (http://www.imagen-europe.com), which examines 2000 adolescents from age 14 to 19 with multiple imaging sessions and neurocognitive assessments (Schumann et al., 2010). Further, the National Institutes of Health has recently approved funding for the most ambitious project to date, the Adolescent Brain Cognitive Development Study (http://www.abcdstudy.org), which will follow 10,000 adolescents starting from ages 9 to 10 for at least 10 years, including imaging and neurocognitive assessment every 2 years and annual assessments of substance use and a multitude of other measures related to development. With the coming influx of longitudinal data, researchers will be able to address many of the gaps in understanding the effects of marijuana and other drugs on brain development and functioning.

6. CONCLUSIONS

Mounting evidence suggests that marijuana use negatively impacts brain structure and function. While there is potential recovery from some of the negative effects of prolonged use, long-term deleterious effects are present and more likely with early age of onset and protracted use. Data from both animal and human models highlight the particularly sensitive period of adolescence for adverse effects of marijuana through the modulation of the neurodevelopmental trajectories. The mechanisms that underlie such modulations are not fully understood and likely result from multiple levels of complex interactions including onset, dose, and duration of marijuana use as well as neurobiological factors including genetic risk. Prolonged marijuana use could result in persistent changes to brain structure and function that underlie the adverse cognitive outcomes associated with heavy use. Future prospective studies with enhanced assessment of marijuana use coupled with MRI assessment prior to and following marijuana use initiation will provide additional clarification of these complex effects of marijuana use on brain structure and function.

REFERENCES

Aarts, E., Roelofs, A., Franke, B., Rijpkema, M., Fernandez, G., Helmich, R. C., & Cools, R. (2010). Striatal dopamine mediates the interface between motivational and cognitive control in humans: Evidence from genetic imaging. *Neuropsychopharmacology*, *35*(9), 1943–1951. http://dx.doi.org/10.1038/npp.2010.68.

Amlien, I. K., Fjell, A. M., Tamnes, C. K., Grydeland, H., Krogsrud, S. K., Chaplin, T. A., ... Walhovd, K. B. (2014). Organizing principles of human cortical development—Thickness and area from 4 to 30 years: Insights from comparative primate neuroanatomy. *Cerebral Cortex*, *26*(1), 257–267. http://dx.doi.org/10.1093/cercor/bhu214.

Arnone, D., Barrick, T. R., Chengappa, S., Mackay, C. E., Clark, C. A., & Abou-Saleh, M. T. (2008). Corpus callosum damage in heavy marijuana use: Preliminary evidence from diffusion tensor tractography and tract-based spatial statistics. *NeuroImage*, *41*(3), 1067–1074. http://dx.doi.org/10.1016/j.neuroimage.2008.02.064.

Ashtari, M., Avants, B., Cyckowski, L., Cervellione, K. L., Roofeh, D., Cook, P., ... Kumra, S. (2011). Medial temporal structures and memory functions in adolescents with heavy cannabis use. *Journal of Psychiatric Research*, *45*(8), 1055–1066. http://dx.doi.org/10.1016/j.jpsychires.2011.01.004.

Ashtari, M., Cervellione, K., Cottone, J., Ardekani, B. A., & Kumra, S. (2009). Diffusion abnormalities in adolescents and young adults with a history of heavy cannabis use. *Journal of Psychiatric Research*, *43*(3), 189–204. http://dx.doi.org/10.1016/j.jpsychires.2008.12.002.

Auer, R., Vittinghoff, E., Yaffe, K., et al. (2016). Association between lifetime marijuana use and cognitive function in middle age: The coronary artery risk development in young adults (cardia) study. *JAMA Internal Medicine*, *176*(3), 352–361. http://dx.doi.org/10.1001/jamainternmed.2015.7841.

Batalla, A., Bhattacharyya, S., Yücel, M., Fusar-Poli, P., Crippa, J. A., Nogué, S., ... Martin-Santos, R. (2013). Structural and functional imaging studies in chronic cannabis users: A systematic review of adolescent and adult findings. *PloS One*, *8*(2), e55821. http://dx.doi.org/10.1371/journal.pone.0055821.

Battistella, G., Fornari, E., Annoni, J.-M., Chtioui, H., Dao, K., Fabritius, M., ... Giroud, C. (2014). Long-term effects of cannabis on brain structure. *Neuropsychopharmacology*, *39*(9), 2041–2048. http://dx.doi.org/10.1038/npp.2014.67.

Bava, S., Frank, L. R., McQueeny, T., Schweinsburg, B. C., Schweinsburg, A. D., & Tapert, S. F. (2009). Altered white matter microstructure in adolescent substance users. *Psychiatry Research: Neuroimaging*, *173*(3), 228–237. http://dx.doi.org/10.1016/j.pscychresns.2009.04.005.

Bava, S., Jacobus, J., Thayer, R. E., & Tapert, S. F. (2013). Longitudinal changes in white matter integrity among adolescent substance users. *Alcoholism, Clinical and Experimental Research*, *37*, E181–E189. http://dx.doi.org/10.1111/j.1530-0277.2012.01920.x.

Bava, S., Thayer, R., Jacobus, J., Ward, M., Jernigan, T. L., & Tapert, S. F. (2010). Longitudinal characterization of white matter maturation during adolescence. *Brain Research*, *1327*, 38–46. http://dx.doi.org/10.1016/j.brainres.2010.02.066.

Becker, M. P., Collins, P. F., Lim, K. O., Muetzel, R. L., & Luciana, M. (2015). Longitudinal changes in white matter microstructure after heavy cannabis use. *Developmental Cognitive Neuroscience*, *16*, 23–35. http://dx.doi.org/10.1016/j.dcn.2015.10.004.

Bhattacharyya, S., Atakan, Z., Martin-Santos, R., Crippa, J. A., & McGuire, P. K. (2012). Neural mechanisms for the cannabinoid modulation of cognition and affect in man:

A critical review of neuroimaging studies. *Current Pharmaceutical Design, 18*(32), 5045–5054. http://dx.doi.org/10.2174/138161212802884636.

Bhattacharyya, S., Morrison, P. D., Fusar-Poli, P., Martin-Santos, R., Borgwardt, S., Winton-Brown, T., … McGuire, P. K. (2010). Opposite effects of delta-9-tetrahydrocannabinol and cannabidiol on human brain function and psychopathology. *Neuropsychopharmacology, 35*(3), 764–774. http://dx.doi.org/10.1038/npp.2009.184.

Bossong, M. G., van Berckel, B. N. M., Boellaard, R., Zuurman, L., Schuit, R. C., Windhorst, A. D., … Kahn, R. S. (2008). [Delta]9-tetrahydrocannabinol induces dopamine release in the human striatum. *Neuropsychopharmacology, 34*(3), 759–766. http://dx.doi.org/10.1038/npp.2008.138.

Brown, S. A., Brumback, T., Tomlinson, K., Cummins, K., Thompson, W. K., Nagel, B. J., … Tapert, S. F. (2015). The National Consortium on Alcohol and NeuroDevelopment in Adolescence (NCANDA): A multisite study of adolescent development and substance use. *Journal of Studies on Alcohol and Drugs, 76*(6), 895–908. http://dx.doi.org/10.15288/jsad.2015.76.895.

Broyd, S. J., van Hell, H. H., Beale, C., Yücel, M., & Solowij, N. (2016). Acute and chronic effects of cannabinoids on human cognition: A systematic review. *Biological Psychiatry, 79*(7), 557–567. http://dx.doi.org/10.1016/j.biopsych.2015.12.002.

Burns, H. D., Van Laere, K., Sanabria-Bohórquez, S., Hamill, T. G., Bormans, G., Eng, W.-S., … Hargreaves, R. J. (2007). [18F]MK-9470, a positron emission tomography (PET) tracer for in vivo human PET brain imaging of the cannabinoid-1 receptor. *Proceedings of the National Academy of Sciences of the United States of America, 104*(23), 9800–9805. http://dx.doi.org/10.1073/pnas.0703472104.

Casey, B. J., Oliveri, M. E., & Insel, T. (2014). A neurodevelopmental perspective on the research domain criteria (RDoC) framework. *Biological Psychiatry, 76*(5), 350–353. http://dx.doi.org/10.1016/j.biopsych.2014.01.006.

Cass, D. K., Flores-Barrera, E., Thomases, D. R., Vital, W. F., Caballero, A., & Tseng, K. Y. (2014). CB1 cannabinoid receptor stimulation during adolescence impairs the maturation of GABA function in the adult rat prefrontal cortex. *Molecular Psychiatry, 19*(5), 536–543. http://dx.doi.org/10.1038/mp.2014.14.

Center for Behavioral Health Statistics and Quality. (2015). *Behavioral health trends in the United States: Results from the 2014 National Survey on Drug Use and Health*. Retrieved from, http://www.samhsa.gov/data/.

Chan, G. C.-K., Hinds, T. R., Impey, S., & Storm, D. R. (1998). Hippocampal neurotoxicity of Δ9-tetrahydrocannabinol. *The Journal of Neuroscience, 18*(14), 5322–5332. Retrieved from, http://www.jneurosci.org/content/18/14/5322.full.

Cheer, J. F., Wassum, K. M., Heien, M. L. A. V., Phillips, P. E. M., & Wightman, R. M. (2004). Cannabinoids enhance subsecond dopamine release in the nucleus accumbens of awake rats. *The Journal of Neuroscience, 24*(18), 4393–4400. http://dx.doi.org/10.1523/jneurosci.0529-04.2004.

Cheetham, A., Allen, N. B., Whittle, S., Simmons, J. G., Yücel, M., & Lubman, D. I. (2012). Orbitofrontal volumes in early adolescence predict initiation of cannabis use: A 4-year longitudinal and prospective study. *Biological Psychiatry, 71*(8), 684–692. http://dx.doi.org/10.1016/j.biopsych.2011.10.029.

Churchwell, J. C., Lopez-Larson, M., & Yurgelun-Todd, D. A. (2010). Altered frontal cortical volume and decision making in adolescent cannabis users. *Frontiers in Psychology, 1*, 225. http://dx.doi.org/10.3389/fpsyg.2010.00225.

Cousijn, J., Wiers, R. W., Ridderinkhof, K. R., van den Brink, W., Veltman, D. J., & Goudriaan, A. E. (2012). Grey matter alterations associated with cannabis use: Results of a VBM study in heavy cannabis users and healthy controls. *NeuroImage, 59*(4), 3845–3851. http://dx.doi.org/10.1016/j.neuroimage.2011.09.046.

Dahl, R. E. (2004). Adolescent brain development: A period of vulnerabilities and opportunities. *Annals of the New York Academy of Sciences*, *1021*(1), 1–22. http://dx.doi.org/10.1196/annals.1308.001.

Demirakca, T., Sartorius, A., Ende, G., Meyer, N., Welzel, H., Skopp, G., … Hermann, D. (2011). Diminished gray matter in the hippocampus of cannabis users: Possible protective effects of cannabidiol. *Drug and Alcohol Dependence*, *114*(2–3), 242–245. http://dx.doi.org/10.1016/j.drugalcdep.2010.09.020.

DiNieri, J. A., & Hurd, Y. L. (2012). Rat models of prenatal and adolescent cannabis exposure. In H. F. Kobeissy (Ed.), *Psychiatric disorders: Methods and protocols* (pp. 231–242). Totowa, NJ: Humana Press.

ElSohly, M. A., Mehmedic, Z., Foster, S., Gon, C., Chandra, S., & Church, J. C. (2016). Changes in cannabis potency over the last two decades (1995–2014)—Analysis of current data in the United States. *Biological Psychiatry*, *79*(7), 613–619. http://dx.doi.org/10.1016/j.biopsych.2016.01.004.

ElSohly, M. A., & Slade, D. (2005). Chemical constituents of marijuana: The complex mixture of natural cannabinoids. *Life Sciences*, *78*(5), 539–548. http://dx.doi.org/10.1016/j.lfs.2005.09.011.

Epstein, K. A., & Kumra, S. (2015a). Altered cortical maturation in adolescent cannabis users with and without schizophrenia. *Schizophrenia Research*, *162*(1–3), 143–152. http://dx.doi.org/10.1016/j.schres.2014.11.029.

Epstein, K. A., & Kumra, S. (2015b). White matter fractional anisotropy over two time points in early onset schizophrenia and adolescent cannabis use disorder: A naturalistic diffusion tensor imaging study. *Psychiatry Research: Neuroimaging*, *232*(1), 34–41. http://dx.doi.org/10.1016/j.pscychresns.2014.10.010.

Filbey, F. M., Aslan, S., Calhoun, V. D., Spence, J. S., Damaraju, E., Caprihan, A., & Segall, J. (2014). Long-term effects of marijuana use on the brain. *Proceedings of the National Academy of Sciences of the United States of America*, *111*(47), 16913–16918. http://dx.doi.org/10.1073/pnas.1415297111.

Filbey, F. M., & DeWitt, S. J. (2012). Cannabis cue-elicited craving and the reward neurocircuitry. *Progress in Neuro-Psychopharmacology and Biological Psychiatry*, *38*(1), 30–35. http://dx.doi.org/10.1016/j.pnpbp.2011.11.001.

Filbey, F. M., McQueeny, T., DeWitt, S. J., & Mishra, V. (2015). Preliminary findings demonstrating latent effects of early adolescent marijuana use onset on cortical architecture. *Developmental Cognitive Neuroscience*, *16*, 16–22. http://dx.doi.org/10.1016/j.dcn.2015.10.001.

Fuhrmann, D., Knoll, L. J., & Blakemore, S.-J. (2015). Adolescence as a sensitive period of brain development. *Trends in Cognitive Sciences*, *19*(10), 558–566. http://dx.doi.org/10.1016/j.tics.2015.07.008.

Gessa, G., Melis, M., Muntoni, A., & Diana, M. (1998). Cannabinoids activate mesolimbic dopamine neurons by an action on cannabinoid CB1 receptors. *European Journal of Pharmacology*, *341*(1), 39–44. http://dx.doi.org/10.1016/S0014-2999(97)01442-8.

Giedd, J. N., Blumenthal, J., Jeffries, N. O., Castellanos, F. X., Liu, H., Zijdenbos, A., … Rapoport, J. L. (1999). Brain development during childhood and adolescence: A longitudinal MRI study. *Nature Neuroscience*, *2*(10), 861–863. http://dx.doi.org/10.1038/13158.

Giedd, J. N., Lalonde, F. M., Celano, M. J., White, S. L., Wallace, G. L., Lee, N. R., & Lenroot, R. K. (2009). Anatomical brain magnetic resonance imaging of typically developing children and adolescents. *Journal of the American Academy of Child and Adolescent Psychiatry*, *48*(5), 465–470. http://dx.doi.org/10.1097/CHI.0b013e31819f2715.

Gilman, J. M., Kuster, J. K., Lee, S., Lee, M. J., Kim, B. W., Makris, N., … Breiter, H. C. (2014). Cannabis use is quantitatively associated with nucleus accumbens and amygdala abnormalities in young adult recreational users. *The Journal of Neuroscience*, *34*(16), 5529–5538. http://dx.doi.org/10.1523/jneurosci.4745-13.2014.

Glass, M., Faull, R. L. M., & Dragunow, M. (1997). Cannabinoid receptors in the human brain: A detailed anatomical and quantitative autoradiographic study in the fetal, neonatal and adult human brain. *Neuroscience*, 77(2), 299–318. http://dx.doi.org/10.1016/S0306-4522(96)00428-9.

Gogtay, N., Giedd, J. N., Lusk, L., Hayashi, K. M., Greenstein, D., Vaituzis, A. C., … Thompson, P. M. (2004). Dynamic mapping of human cortical development during childhood through early adulthood. *Proceedings of the National Academy of Sciences of the United States of America*, *101*(21), 8174–8179. http://dx.doi.org/10.1073/pnas.0402680101.

Gruber, S. A., Dahlgren, M. K., Sagar, K. A., Gönenç, A., & Lukas, S. E. (2014). Worth the wait: Effects of age of onset of marijuana use on white matter and impulsivity. *Psychopharmacology*, *231*(8), 1455–1465. http://dx.doi.org/10.1007/s00213-013-3326-z.

Gruber, S. A., Silveri, M. M., Dahlgren, M. K., & Yurgelun-Todd, D. (2011). Why so impulsive? White matter alterations are associated with impulsivity in chronic marijuana smokers. *Experimental and Clinical Psychopharmacology*, *19*(3), 231–242. http://dx.doi.org/10.1037/a0023034.

Harding, I. H., Solowij, N., Harrison, B. J., Takagi, M., Lorenzetti, V., Lubman, D. I., … Yucel, M. (2012). Functional connectivity in brain networks underlying cognitive control in chronic cannabis users. *Neuropsychopharmacology*, *37*(8), 1923–1933. http://dx.doi.org/10.1038/npp.2012.39.

Hartman, R. L., Brown, T. L., Milavetz, G., Spurgin, A., Gorelick, D. A., Gaffney, G., & Huestis, M. A. (2015). Controlled vaporized cannabis, with and without alcohol: Subjective effects and oral fluid-blood cannabinoid relationships. *Drug Testing and Analysis*. http://dx.doi.org/10.1002/dta.1839. (online early view).

Hartman, R. L., Brown, T. L., Milavetz, G., Spurgin, A., Gorelick, D. A., Gaffney, G. R., & Huestis, M. A. (2016). Effect of blood collection time on measured Δ9-tetrahydrocannabinol concentrations: Implications for driving interpretation and drug policy. *Clinical Chemistry*, *62*(2), 367–377. http://dx.doi.org/10.1373/clinchem.2015.248492.

Hester, R., Nestor, L., & Garavan, H. (2009). Impaired error awareness and anterior cingulate cortex hypoactivity in chronic cannabis users. *Neuropsychopharmacology*, *34*(11), 2450–2458. http://dx.doi.org/10.1038/npp.2009.67.

Hirvonen, J., Goodwin, R. S., Li, C. T., Terry, G. E., Zoghbi, S. S., Morse, C., … Innis, R. B. (2012). Reversible and regionally selective downregulation of brain cannabinoid CB(1) receptors in chronic daily cannabis smokers. *Molecular Psychiatry*, *17*(6), 642–649. http://dx.doi.org/10.1038/mp.2011.82.

Hurd, Y. L., Michaelides, M., Miller, M. L., & Jutras-Aswad, D. (2014). Trajectory of adolescent cannabis use on addiction vulnerability. *Neuropharmacology*, *76*(Pt. B), 416–424. http://dx.doi.org/10.1016/j.neuropharm.2013.07.028.

Huttenlocher, P. R., & Dabholkar, A. S. (1997). Regional differences in synaptogenesis in human cerebral cortex. *The Journal of Comparative Neurology*, *387*(2), 167–178. http://dx.doi.org/10.1002/(SICI)1096-9861(19971020)387:2<167::AID-CNE1>3.0.CO;2-Z.

Jackson, N. J., Isen, J. D., Khoddam, R., Irons, D., Tuvblad, C., Iacono, W. G., … Baker, L. A. (2016). Impact of adolescent marijuana use on intelligence: Results from two longitudinal twin studies. *Proceedings of the National Academy of Sciences of the United States of America*, *113*(5), E500–E508. http://dx.doi.org/10.1073/pnas.1516648113.

Jacobus, J., Bava, S., Cohen-Zion, M., Mahmood, O., & Tapert, S. F. (2009). Functional consequences of marijuana use in adolescents. *Pharmacology, Biochemistry, and Behavior*, *92*(4), 559–565. http://dx.doi.org/10.1016/j.pbb.2009.04.001.

Jacobus, J., McQueeny, T., Bava, S., Schweinsburg, B. C., Frank, L. R., Yang, T. T., & Tapert, S. F. (2009). White matter integrity in adolescents with histories of marijuana use and binge drinking. *Neurotoxicology and Teratology, 31*(6), 349–355. http://dx.doi.org/10.1016/j.ntt.2009.07.006.

Jacobus, J., Squeglia, L. M., Bava, S., & Tapert, S. F. (2013a). White matter characterization of adolescent binge drinking with and without co-occurring marijuana use: A 3-year investigation. *Psychiatry Research: Neuroimaging, 214*(3), 374–381. http://dx.doi.org/10.1016/j.pscychresns.2013.07.014.

Jacobus, J., Squeglia, L. M., Infante, M. A., Bava, S., & Tapert, S. F. (2013b). White matter integrity pre- and post marijuana and alcohol initiation in adolescence. *Brain Sciences, 3*(1), 396–414. http://dx.doi.org/10.3390/brainsci3010396.

Jacobus, J., Squeglia, L. M., Meruelo, A. D., Castro, N., Brumback, T., Giedd, J. N., & Tapert, S. F. (2015). Cortical thickness in adolescent marijuana and alcohol users: A three-year prospective study from adolescence to young adulthood. *Developmental Cognitive Neuroscience, 16*, 101–109. http://dx.doi.org/10.1016/j.dcn.2015.04.006.

Jacobus, J., Thayer, R. E., Trim, R. S., Bava, S., Frank, L. R., & Tapert, S. F. (2013). White matter integrity, substance use, and risk taking in adolescence. *Psychology of Addictive Behaviors, 27*(2), 431–442. http://dx.doi.org/10.1037/a0028235.

Johnston, L. D., O'Malley, P. M., Miech, R. A., Bachman, J. G., & Schulenberg, J. E. (2015). *Monitoring the future national survey results on drug use: 2014 Overview, key findings on adolescent drug use.* Ann Arbor: Institute for Social Research, The University of Michigan.

Koepp, M. J., Gunn, R. N., Lawrence, A. D., Cunningham, V. J., Dagher, A., Jones, T., ... Grasby, P. M. (1998). Evidence for striatal dopamine release during a video game. *Nature, 393*(6682), 266–268. http://dx.doi.org/10.1038/30498.

Kolb, B., Gorny, G., Limebeer, C. L., & Parker, L. A. (2006). Chronic treatment with Δ-9-tetrahydrocannabinol alters the structure of neurons in the nucleus accumbens shell and medial prefrontal cortex of rats. *Synapse, 60*(6), 429–436. http://dx.doi.org/10.1002/syn.20313.

Koob, G. F., & Le Moal, M. (2001). Drug addiction, dysregulation of reward, and allostasis. *Neuropsychopharmacology, 24*(2), 97–129.

Koob, G. F., & Volkow, N. D. (2010). Neurocircuitry of addiction. *Neuropsychopharmacology, 35*(1), 217–238. http://dx.doi.org/10.1038/npp.2009.110.

Kook, G. F., & Weiss, F. (1992). Neuropharmacology of cocaine and ethanol dependence. *Recent Developments in Alcoholism, 10*, 201–233.

Lebel, C., Gee, M., Camicioli, R., Wieler, M., Martin, W., & Beaulieu, C. (2012). Diffusion tensor imaging of white matter tract evolution over the lifespan. *NeuroImage, 60*(1), 340–352. http://dx.doi.org/10.1016/j.neuroimage.2011.11.094.

Lopez-Larson, M. P., Bogorodzki, P., Rogowska, J., McGlade, E., King, J. B., Terry, J., & Yurgelun-Todd, D. (2011). Altered prefrontal and insular cortical thickness in adolescent marijuana users. *Behavioural Brain Research, 220*(1), 164–172. http://dx.doi.org/10.1016/j.bbr.2011.02.001.

Lopez-Larson, M. P., Rogowska, J., & Yurgelun-Todd, D. (2015). Aberrant orbitofrontal connectivity in marijuana smoking adolescents. *Developmental Cognitive Neuroscience, 16*, 54–62. http://dx.doi.org/10.1016/j.dcn.2015.08.002.

Lorenzetti, V., Solowij, N., Fornito, A., Ian Lubman, D., & Yucel, M. (2014). The association between regular cannabis exposure and alterations of human brain morphology: An updated review of the literature. *Current Pharmaceutical Design, 20*(13), 2138–2167. http://dx.doi.org/10.2174/13816128113199990435.

Lorenzetti, V., Solowij, N., Whittle, S., Fornito, A., Lubman, D. I., Pantelis, C., & Yücel, M. (2015). Gross morphological brain changes with chronic, heavy cannabis use. *The British Journal of Psychiatry, 206*(1), 77–78. http://dx.doi.org/10.1192/bjp.bp.114.151407.

Lorenzetti, V., Solowij, N., & Yücel, M. (2016). The role of cannabinoids on neuroanatomical alterations in cannabis users. *Biological Psychiatry*, *79*(7), e17–e31. http://dx.doi.org/10.1016/j.biopsych.2015.11.013.
Lubman, D. I., Cheetham, A., & Yücel, M. (2015). Cannabis and adolescent brain development. *Pharmacology & Therapeutics*, *148*, 1–16. http://dx.doi.org/10.1016/j.pharmthera.2014.11.009.
Luciana, M. (2013). Adolescent brain development in normality and psychopathology. *Development and Psychopathology*, *25*(25th Anniversary Special Issue 4 Pt. 2), 1325–1345. http://dx.doi.org/10.1017/S0954579413000643.
Martín-Santos, R., Fagundo, A. B., Crippa, J. A., Atakan, Z., Bhattacharyya, S., Allen, P., … McGuire, P. (2010). Neuroimaging in cannabis use: A systematic review of the literature. *Psychological Medicine*, *40*(3), 383–398. http://dx.doi.org/10.1017/S0033291709990729.
Mato, S., Chevaleyre, V., Robbe, D., Pazos, A., Castillo, P. E., & Manzoni, O. J. (2004). A single in-vivo exposure to [Delta]9THC blocks endocannabinoid-mediated synaptic plasticity. *Nature Neuroscience*, 7(6), 585–586. http://dx.doi.org/10.1038/nn1251.
Matochik, J. A., Eldreth, D. A., Cadet, J.-L., & Bolla, K. I. (2005). Altered brain tissue composition in heavy marijuana users. *Drug and Alcohol Dependence*, 77(1), 23–30. http://dx.doi.org/10.1016/j.drugalcdep.2004.06.011.
Medina, K. L., Nagel, B. J., & Tapert, S. F. (2010). Abnormal cerebellar morphometry in abstinent adolescent marijuana users. *Psychiatry Research*, *182*(2), 152–159. http://dx.doi.org/10.1016/j.pscychresns.2009.12.004.
Meier, M. H., Caspi, A., Ambler, A., Harrington, H., Houts, R., Keefe, R. S. E., … Moffitt, T. E. (2012). Persistent cannabis users show neuropsychological decline from childhood to midlife. *Proceedings of the National Academy of Sciences of the United States of America*, *109*(40), E2657–E2664. http://dx.doi.org/10.1073/pnas.1206820109.
Nestor, L., Hester, R., & Garavan, H. (2010). Increased ventral striatal BOLD activity during non-drug reward anticipation in cannabis users. *NeuroImage*, *49*(1), 1133–1143. http://dx.doi.org/10.1016/j.neuroimage.2009.07.022.
Nestor, L., Roberts, G., Garavan, H., & Hester, R. (2008). Deficits in learning and memory: Parahippocampal hyperactivity and frontocortical hypoactivity in cannabis users. *NeuroImage*, *40*(3), 1328–1339. http://dx.doi.org/10.1016/j.neuroimage.2007.12.059.
Orr, C., Morioka, R., Behan, B., Datwani, S., Doucet, M., Ivanovic, J., … Garavan, H. (2013). Altered resting-state connectivity in adolescent cannabis users. *The American Journal of Drug and Alcohol Abuse*, *39*(6), 372–381. http://dx.doi.org/10.3109/00952990.2013.848213.
Padula, C., Schweinsburg, A., & Tapert, S. (2007). Spatial working memory performance and fMRI activation interaction in abstinent adolescent marijuana users. *Psychology of Addictive Behaviors*, *21*(4), 478–487. http://dx.doi.org/10.1037/0893-164X.21.4.478.
Pfefferbaum, A., Rohlfing, T., Pohl, K. M., Lane, B., Chu, W., Kwon, D., … Sullivan, E. V. (2015). Adolescent development of cortical and white matter structure in the NCANDA sample: Role of sex, ethnicity, puberty, and alcohol drinking. *Cerebral Cortex*, http://dx.doi.org/10.1093/cercor/bhv205. (online early view).
Quinn, H. R., Matsumoto, I., Callaghan, P. D., Long, L. E., Arnold, J. C., Gunasekaran, N., … McGregor, I. S. (2007). Adolescent rats find repeated [Delta]9-THC less aversive than adult rats but display greater residual cognitive deficits and changes in hippocampal protein expression following exposure. *Neuropsychopharmacology*, *33*(5), 1113–1126. http://dx.doi.org/10.1038/sj.npp.1301475.
Ramaekers, J., Kauert, G., Theunissen, E., Toennes, S., & Moeller, M. (2009). Neurocognitive performance during acute THC intoxication in heavy and occasional

cannabis users. *Journal of Psychopharmacology*, *23*(3), 266–277. http://dx.doi.org/10.1177/0269881108092393.

Ranganathan, M., & D'Souza, D. C. (2006). The acute effects of cannabinoids on memory in humans: A review. *Psychopharmacology*, *188*(4), 425–444. http://dx.doi.org/10.1007/s00213-006-0508-y.

Raver, S. M., & Keller, A. (2014). Permanent suppression of cortical oscillations in mice after adolescent exposure to cannabinoids: Receptor mechanisms. *Neuropharmacology*, *86*, 161–173. http://dx.doi.org/10.1016/j.neuropharm.2014.07.006.

Raznahan, A., Shaw, P., Lalonde, F., Stockman, M., Wallace, G. L., Greenstein, D., … Giedd, J. N. (2011). How does your cortex grow? *The Journal of Neuroscience*, *31*(19), 7174–7177. http://dx.doi.org/10.1523/jneurosci.0054-11.2011.

Renard, J., Vitalis, T., Rame, M., Krebs, M.-O., Lenkei, Z., Le Pen, G., & Jay, T. M. (2016). Chronic cannabinoid exposure during adolescence leads to long-term structural and functional changes in the prefrontal cortex. *European Neuropsychopharmacology*, *26*(1), 55–64. http://dx.doi.org/10.1016/j.euroneuro.2015.11.005.

Robbin, T. W., & Everitt, B. J. (2002). Limbic-striatal memory system and drug addiction. *Neurobiology of Learning and Memory*, *78*(3), 625–636.

Rubino, T., & Parolaro, D. (2016). The impact of exposure to cannabinoids in adolescence: Insights from animal models. *Biological Psychiatry*, *79*(7), 578–585. http://dx.doi.org/10.1016/j.biopsych.2015.07.024.

Rubino, T., Realini, N., Braida, D., Guidi, S., Capurro, V., Viganò, D., … Parolaro, D. (2009). Changes in hippocampal morphology and neuroplasticity induced by adolescent THC treatment are associated with cognitive impairment in adulthood. *Hippocampus*, *19*(8), 763–772. http://dx.doi.org/10.1002/hipo.20554.

Sagar, K. A., Dahlgren, M. K., Gönenç, A., Racine, M. T., Dreman, M. W., & Gruber, S. A. (2015). The impact of initiation: Early onset marijuana smokers demonstrate altered Stroop performance and brain activation. *Developmental Cognitive Neuroscience*, *16*, 84–92. http://dx.doi.org/10.1016/j.dcn.2015.03.003.

SAMHSA. (2014). *Results from the 2013 national survey on drug use and health: Summary of national findings*. Rockville, MD: US Department of Health and Human Services, Substance Abuse and Mental Health Services Administration.

Schacht, J. P., Hutchison, K. E., & Filbey, F. M. (2012). Associations between cannabinoid receptor-1 (CNR1) variation and hippocampus and amygdala volumes in heavy cannabis users. *Neuropsychopharmacology*, *37*(11), 2368–2376. http://dx.doi.org/10.1038/npp.2012.92.

Schreiner, A., & Dunn, M. (2012). Residual effects of cannabis use on neurocognitive performance after prolonged abstinence: A meta-analysis. *Experimental and Clinical Psychopharmacology*, *20*(5), 420–429. http://dx.doi.org/10.1037/a0029117.

Schumann, G., Loth, E., Banaschewski, T., Barbot, A., Barker, G., Buchel, C., … Struve, M. (2010). The IMAGEN study: Reinforcement-related behaviour in normal brain function and psychopathology. *Molecular Psychiatry*, *15*(12), 1128–1139. http://dx.doi.org/10.1038/mp.2010.4.

Schweinsburg, A. D., McQueeny, T., Nagel, B. J., Eyler, L. T., & Tapert, S. F. (2010). A preliminary study of functional magnetic resonance imaging response during verbal encoding among adolescent binge drinkers. *Alcohol*, *44*(1), 111–117. Retrieved from PMCID: PMC2845466.

Schweinsburg, A. D., Nagel, B. J., Schweinsburg, B. C., Park, A., Theilmann, R. J., & Tapert, S. F. (2008). Abstinent adolescent marijuana users show altered fMRI response during spatial working memory. *Psychiatry Research: Neuroimaging*, *163*(1), 40–51. http://dx.doi.org/10.1016/j.pscychresns.2007.04.018.

Schweinsburg, A. D., Schweinsburg, B. C., Cheung, E. H., Brown, G. G., Brown, S. A., & Tapert, S. F. (2005). fMRI response to spatial working memory in adolescents with comorbid marijuana and alcohol use disorders. *Drug and Alcohol Dependence*, *79*(2), 201–210. http://dx.doi.org/10.1016/j.drugalcdep.2005.01.009.

Schweinsburg, A. D., Schweinsburg, B. C., Medina, K. L., McQueeny, T., Brown, S. A., & Tapert, S. F. (2010). The influence of recency of use on fMRI response during spatial working memory in adolescent marijuana users. *Journal of Psychoactive Drugs*, *42*(3), 401–412. http://dx.doi.org/10.1080/02791072.2010.10400703.

Selemon, L. D. (2013). A role for synaptic plasticity in the adolescent development of executive function. *Translational Psychiatry*, *3*, e238. http://dx.doi.org/10.1038/tp.2013.7.

Shaw, P., Kabani, N. J., Lerch, J. P., Eckstrand, K., Lenroot, R., Gogtay, N., … Wise, S. P. (2008). Neurodevelopmental trajectories of the human cerebral cortex. *The Journal of Neuroscience*, *28*(14), 3586–3594. http://dx.doi.org/10.1523/jneurosci.5309-07.2008.

Sim-Selley, L. J. (2003). Regulation of cannabinoid CB1 receptors in the central nervous system by chronic cannabinoids. *Critical Reviews in Neurobiology*, *15*(2), 30. http://dx.doi.org/10.1615/CritRevNeurobiol.v15.i2.10.

Smith, A., Longo, C., Fried, P., Hogan, M., & Cameron, I. (2010). Effects of marijuana on visuospatial working memory: An fMRI study in young adults. *Psychopharmacology*, *210*(3), 429–438. http://dx.doi.org/10.1007/s00213-010-1841-8.

Solowij, N., Yücel, M., Respondek, C., Whittle, S., Lindsay, E., Pantelis, C., & Lubman, D. I. (2011). Cerebellar white-matter changes in cannabis users with and without schizophrenia. *Psychological Medicine*, *41*(11), 2349–2359. http://dx.doi.org/10.1017/S003329171100050X.

Sowell, E. R., Thompson, P. M., Holmes, C. J., Jernigan, T. L., & Toga, A. W. (1999). In vivo evidence for post-adolescent brain maturation in frontal and striatal regions. *Nature Neuroscience*, *2*(10), 859–861.

Tapert, S., Schweinsburg, A., Drummond, S. A., Paulus, M., Brown, S., Yang, T., & Frank, L. (2007). Functional MRI of inhibitory processing in abstinent adolescent marijuana users. *Psychopharmacology*, *194*(2), 173–183. http://dx.doi.org/10.1007/s00213-007-0823-y.

Thatcher, D. L., Pajtek, S., Chung, T., Terwilliger, R. A., & Clark, D. B. (2010). Gender differences in the relationship between white matter organization and adolescent substance use disorders. *Drug and Alcohol Dependence*, *110*(1–2), 55–61. http://dx.doi.org/10.1016/j.drugalcdep.2010.02.004.

Toga, A. W., Thompson, P. M., & Sowell, E. R. (2006). Mapping brain maturation. *Trends in Neurosciences*, *29*(3), 148–159. http://dx.doi.org/10.1016/j.tins.2006.01.007.

UNODC. (2014). *World drug report 2014 (Sales No. E.14.XI.7)*. Vienna, Austria: United Nations Office on Drugs and Crime. Retrieved from, http://www.unodc.org/documents/wdr2014/World_Drug_Report_2014_web.pdf.

Urban, N. B., Slifstein, M., Meda, S., Xu, X., Ayoub, R., Medina, O., … Abi-Dargham, A. (2012). Imaging human reward processing with positron emission tomography and functional magnetic resonance imaging. *Psychopharmacology*, *221*(1), 67–77. http://dx.doi.org/10.1007/s00213-011-2543-6.

van Hell, H. H., Jager, G., Bossong, M. G., Brouwer, A., Jansma, J. M., Zuurman, L., … Ramsey, N. F. (2012). Involvement of the endocannabinoid system in reward processing in the human brain. *Psychopharmacology*, *219*(4), 981–990. http://dx.doi.org/10.1007/s00213-011-2428-8.

van Hell, H. H., Vink, M., Ossewaarde, L., Jager, G., Kahn, R. S., & Ramsey, N. F. (2010). Chronic effects of cannabis use on the human reward system: An fMRI study. *European Neuropsychopharmacology*, *20*(3), 153–163. http://dx.doi.org/10.1016/j.euroneuro.2009.11.010.

Van Waes, V., Beverley, J., Siman, H., Tseng, K. Y., & Steiner, H. (2012). CB1 cannabinoid receptor expression in the striatum: Association with corticostriatal circuits and developmental regulation. *Frontiers in Pharmacology 3.* http://dx.doi.org/10.3389/fphar.2012.00021.

Verdurand, M., Nguyen, V., Stark, D., Zahra, D., Gregoire, M.-C., Greguric, I., & Zavitsanou, K. (2011). Comparison of cannabinoid CB(1) receptor binding in adolescent and adult rats: A positron emission tomography study using [(18)F]MK-9470. *International Journal of Molecular Imaging, 2011,* 548123. http://dx.doi.org/10.1155/2011/548123.

Volkow, N. D., & Baler, R. D. (2014). Addiction science: Uncovering neurobiological complexity. *Neuropharmacology, 76*(Pt. B), 235–249. http://dx.doi.org/10.1016/j.neuropharm.2013.05.007.

Volkow, N. D., Baler, R. D., Compton, W. M., & Weiss, S. R. B. (2014). Adverse health effects of marijuana use. *New England Journal of Medicine, 370*(23), 2219–2227. http://dx.doi.org/10.1056/NEJMra1402309.

Volkow, N. D., Koob, G. F., & McLellan, A. T. (2016). Neurobiologic advances from the brain disease model of addiction. *New England Journal of Medicine, 374*(4), 363–371. http://dx.doi.org/10.1056/NEJMra1511480.

Volkow, N. D., Swanson, J. M., Evins, A. E., DeLisi, L. E., Meier, M. H., Gonzalez, R., ... Baler, R. (2016). Effects of cannabis use on human behavior, including cognition, motivation, and psychosis: A review. *JAMA Psychiatry, 73*(3), 292–297. http://dx.doi.org/10.1001/jamapsychiatry.2015.3278.

Walhovd, K. B., Fjell, A. M., Giedd, J., Dale, A. M., & Brown, T. T. (2016). Through thick and thin: A need to reconcile contradictory results on trajectories in human cortical development. *Cerebral Cortex,* http://dx.doi.org/10.1093/cercor/bhv301. (online early access).

Weiland, B. J., Thayer, R. E., Depue, B. E., Sabbineni, A., Bryan, A. D., & Hutchison, K. E. (2015). Daily marijuana use is not associated with brain morphometric measures in adolescents or adults. *The Journal of Neuroscience, 35*(4), 1505–1512. http://dx.doi.org/10.1523/jneurosci.2946-14.2015.

Wesley, M. J., Hanlon, C. A., & Porrino, L. J. (2011). Poor decision-making by chronic marijuana users is associated with decreased functional responsiveness to negative consequences. *Psychiatry Research: Neuroimaging, 191*(1), 51–59. http://dx.doi.org/10.1016/j.pscychresns.2010.10.002.

Yip, S. W., DeVito, E. E., Kober, H., Worhunsky, P. D., Carroll, K. M., & Potenza, M. N. (2014). Pretreatment measures of brain structure and reward-processing brain function in cannabis dependence: An exploratory study of relationships with abstinence during behavioral treatment. *Drug and Alcohol Dependence, 140,* 33–41. http://dx.doi.org/10.1016/j.drugalcdep.2014.03.031.

Yucel, M., Solowij, N., Respondek, C., Whittle, S., Fornito, A., Pantelis, C., & Lubman, D. I. (2008). Regional brain abnormalities associated with long-term heavy cannabis use. *Archives of General Psychiatry, 65*(6), 694–701. http://dx.doi.org/10.1001/archpsyc.65.6.694.

Zalesky, A., Solowij, N., Yücel, M., Lubman, D. I., Takagi, M., Harding, I. H., ... Seal, M. (2012). Effect of long-term cannabis use on axonal fibre connectivity. *Brain, 135*(7), 2245–2255. http://dx.doi.org/10.3109/10826084.2010.482443.

CHAPTER THREE

Neurobiological Basis of Hypersexuality

S. Kühn*,†,1, J. Gallinat*
*University Clinic Hamburg-Eppendorf, Clinic and Polyclinic for Psychiatry and Psychotherapy, Hamburg, Germany
†Center for Lifespan Psychology, Max Planck Institute for Human Development, Berlin, Germany
[1]Corresponding author: e-mail address: kuehn@mpib-berlin.mpg.de

Contents

Abstract

Until now, hypersexuality has not found entry into the common diagnostic classification systems. However it is a frequently discussed phenomenon consisting of excessive sexual appetite that is maladaptive for the individual. Initial studies investigated the neurobiological underpinnings of hypersexuality, but current literature is still insufficient to draw unequivocal conclusions. In the present review, we summarize and discuss findings from various perspectives: neuroimaging and lesion studies, studies on other neurological disorders that are sometimes accompanied by hypersexuality, neuropharmacological evidence, genetic as well as animal studies. Taken together, the evidence seems to imply that alterations in the frontal lobe, amygdala, hippocampus, hypothalamus, septum, and brain regions that process reward play a prominent role in the emergence of hypersexuality. Genetic studies and neuropharmacological treatment approaches point at an involvement of the dopaminergic system.

International Review of Neurobiology, Volume 129
ISSN 0074-7742
http://dx.doi.org/10.1016/bs.irn.2016.04.002

1. DEFINITION OF HYPERSEXUALITY

Different terms have been used to describe the phenomenon of persistent, socially deviant sexual behavior accompanied by excessive sexual appetite that is maladaptive for the individual. Most frequently found are the terms "hypersexuality," "compulsive sexual behavior," and "sex addiction." Other terms that have been introduced for this condition are "Don Juanism" or "satyriasis" in men and "nymphomania" in women. We will in the following use the term "hypersexuality" since this terminology does not imply a theoretical bias toward an association with obsessive–compulsive disorder—as may be suspected in using the term "compulsive sexual behavior"—nor with substance addictions, as implicated in the term "sex addiction." Moreover, whether hypersexuality should be considered in the new Diagnostic and Statistical Manual of Mental Disorders, Fifth Edition (DSM-5) was discussed using this nomination. The American Psychiatric Association decided against introducing hypersexual disorder as a distinct diagnostic category (Reid & Kafka, 2014), and hypersexuality was not included in the DSM-5 mostly due to a lack of research on valid diagnostic criteria.

In terms of quantifying hypersexuality, Kinsey introduced the concept of total sexual outlet, under which he subsumed the total number of weekly orgasms, independently of how it was achieved be it by masturbation, intercourse, etc. (Kinsey, Pomeroy, & Martin, 1948). Data suggest that only 7.6% of American males below 30 years report more than seven weekly sexual outlets for at least 5 years. Based on these empirical quantities, Kafka proposed to characterize hypersexuality as more than seven total sexual outlets per week (Kafka, 1997).

In the present review, we will summarize the neurobiological evidence that has accumulated on hypersexuality as well as on sexual arousal in general and excessive pornography consumption in particular.

2. PREVALENCE AND COMORBIDITY OF HYPERSEXUALITY

The mean age of onset of hypersexuality was estimated at 18.7 years in sexually active men (Kafka & Hennen, 2003) with an average duration of 12.3 years. Treatment was on average only sought at an average age of 37. Research suggests that women are less vulnerable to hypersexuality than men. The sex ratio has been estimated to be 5:1 (male:female)

(Kuzma & Black, 2008). Generally hypersexuality is estimated to affect 3–6% of the population. Frequently observed comorbidities of hypersexuality include mood disorders (72%, Kafka & Hennen, 2002), anxiety disorders (38%, Kafka & Hennen, 2002), substance abuse (40%, Kafka & Hennen, 2002; 71%, Raymond, Coleman, & Miner, 2003; 64%, Black, Kehrberg, Flumerfelt, & Schlosser, 1997), personality disorders (17%, Carpenter, Reid, Garos, & Najavits, 2013), and obsessive–compulsive disorders (<15%, Kingston & Firestone, 2008; Raymond et al., 2003). In line with the comorbidity with substance abuse, 79% of self-reported swingers also report drug use for recreational purposes, including alcohol (Spauwen, Niekamp, Hoebe, & Dukers-Muijrers, 2015). Moreover, recreational drug use (excluding alcohol intake) is linked to high-risk sexual behavior. Likewise psychostimulant and heroin users are more likely to engage in high-risk sexual behaviors (Jia et al., 2013).

3. HYPERSEXUALITY AS AN OBSESSIVE–COMPULSIVE, IMPULSE, OR ADDICTION DISORDER

The phenomenon of hypersexuality has sometimes been classified as an obsessive–compulsive disorder, sometimes as an impulse disorder, and sometimes as an addiction disorder in terms of its etiology.

Evidence for a classification of hypersexuality as an obsessive–compulsive disorder may stem from the fact that both phenomena involve intrusive thoughts as well as compulsions. Some reports suggest that these compulsions are sometimes enacted with the goal to reduce anxiety. Another interesting aspect is that both disorders seem to respond to pharmacological treatment with selective serotonin reuptake inhibitors (SSRIs), evidence to support common pharmacology between hypersexuality and obsessive–compulsive disorder (Mick & Hollander, 2006). However, the comorbidity between the two phenomena seems to be fairly low (15%) (Kingston & Firestone, 2008; Raymond et al., 2003).

A resemblance to impulse control disorders may be seen in the fact that people suffering from hypersexuality may be unable to resist temptation (Barth & Kinder, 1987).

Garcia and Thibaut have argued that hypersexuality should be classified as an addiction disorder (Garcia & Thibaut, 2010). Their reasoning is based on the fact that both hypersexuality and substance addiction involve an escalation of consumption as the disease develops, withdrawal symptoms such as depression or anxiety, and difficulty in reducing or stopping the behavior.

Indeed, individuals suffering from hypersexuality continue their behavior despite the potential of or experience of adverse consequences. Moreover, the amount of time spent having an outlet often results in a reduction of time spent with family, friends, and other healthy activities. These features appear to characterize both substance addictions and hypersexuality. Although the exact numbers vary between studies, comorbidity between hypersexuality and substance addictions is high (between 40% and 71%).

4. NEUROIMAGING CORRELATES OF HYPERSEXUALITY

Multiple studies have investigated the neural correlates of sexual arousal in response to visual erotic stimuli in comparison to neutral stimuli using functional magnetic resonance imaging (fMRI). In a meta-analysis on multiple neuroimaging studies investigating brain responses to visual erotic cues conducted in male heterosexuals, we found convergence across studies in BOLD activation in several regions including hypothalamus, thalamus, amygdala, anterior cingulate gyrus (ACC), insula, fusiform gyrus, precentral gyrus, parietal cortex, and occipital cortex (Kühn & Gallinat, 2011a) (Fig. 1). In studies that reported brain responses associated with a physiological marker of sexual arousal (eg, penile tumescence), we found consistent activation across studies in hypothalamus, thalamus, bilateral insula, ACC, postcentral gyrus, and occipital gyrus.

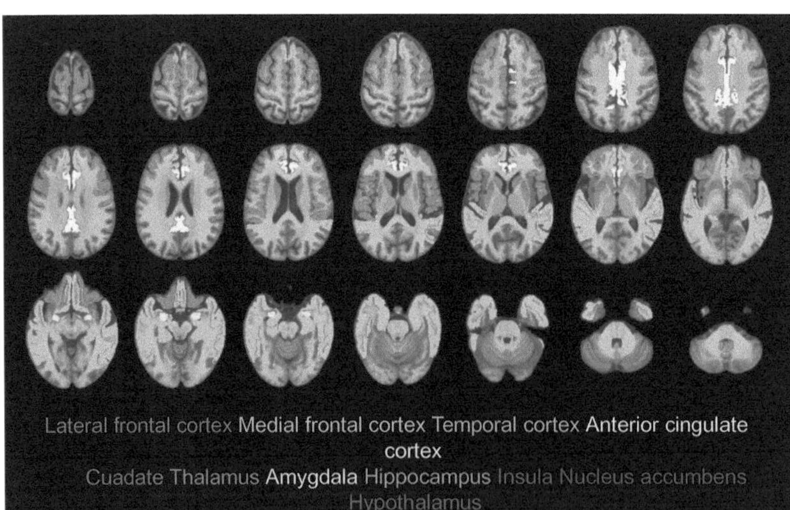

Fig. 1 Regions potentially involved in hypersexual behaviors (septum not shown).

In studies in which brain activity was monitored during orgasm for men and women, activation was reported in dopaminergic pathways originating from the ventral tegmentum (VTA) (Holstege et al., 2003) to the nucleus accumbens (Komisaruk et al., 2004; Komisaruk, Wise, Frangos, Birbano, & Allen, 2011). Activity was also observed in cerebellum and the ACC (Holstege et al., 2003; Komisaruk et al., 2004, 2011). In women only, frontal cortical brain activation was observed during orgasm (Komisaruk & Whipple, 2005).

In a cue-reactivity study on cocaine-addicted patients, individuals were presented with visual cues related to either cocaine or sex (Childress et al., 2008). Interestingly, the results revealed similar brain regions to be activated during drug-related and sex-related cues located in the reward network and the limbic system, namely in VTA, amygdala, nucleus accumbens, orbitofrontal, and insular cortex. Others have remarked a similarity in the cerebral activation profile in response to sexual stimuli and love and attachment (Frascella, Potenza, Brown, & Childress, 2010).

Only a single study to date has, to our knowledge, investigated differences in brain activation between participants with and without hypersexuality during a cue-reactivity fMRI task (Voon et al., 2014). The authors report higher ACC, ventral striatal, and amygdala activity in individuals with hypersexuality compared with those without. The areas activated overlap with brain regions that we identified in a meta-analysis to be consistently activated in drug-craving paradigms across different types of substance addictions (Kühn & Gallinat, 2011b). This regional similarity offers further support for the hypothesis that hypersexuality may indeed be most similar to addiction disorders. The study by Voon and colleagues also revealed that high functional connectivity of the ACC–striatal–amygdala network was associated with subjectively reported sexual desire ("wanting" in reply to the question "How much did this increase your sexual desire?" not "liking" assessed by the question "How much did you like this video?") to a higher degree in patients with hypersexuality. Moreover, the patients with hypersexuality reported higher levels of "wanting" but not of "liking." This dissociation between "wanting" and "liking" has been hypothesized to occur once a certain behavior becomes an addiction within the framework of the so-called incentive-salience theory of addiction (Robinson & Berridge, 2008).

In an electroencephalography study on participants complaining about difficulties in controlling their consumption of internet pornography, event-related potentials (ERPs), namely P300 amplitudes in response to emotional and sexual cues, were tested for an association with questionnaire scores assessing hypersexuality and sexual desire (wanting) (Steele, Staley, Fong, & Prause, 2013). The P300 has been related to attentional processes and is in part generated in the ACC. The authors interpret the absence of a correlation between questionnaire scores and ERP amplitudes as a failure to support previous models of hypersexuality. This conclusion has been criticized as unjustified by others (Love, Laier, Brand, Hatch, & Hajela, 2015; Watts & Hilton, 2011).

In a recent study by our group, we recruited healthy male participants and associated their self-reported hours spent with pornographic material with their fMRI response to sexual pictures as well as with their brain morphology (Kühn & Gallinat, 2014). The more hours participants reported consuming pornography, the smaller the BOLD response in left putamen in response to sexual images. Moreover, we found that more hours spent watching pornography was associated with smaller gray matter volume in the striatum, more precisely in the right caudate reaching into the ventral putamen. We speculate that the brain structural volume deficit may reflect the results of tolerance after desensitization to sexual stimuli. The discrepancy between the results reported by Voon and colleagues could be due to the fact that our participants were recruited from the general population and were not diagnosed as suffering from hypersexuality. However, it may well be that still pictures of pornographic content (in contrast to videos as used in the study by Voon) may not satisfy today's video porn viewers, as suggested by Love and colleagues (2015). In terms of functional connectivity, we found that participants who consumed more pornography showed less connectivity between the right caudate (where the volume was found to be smaller) and left dorsolateral prefrontal cortex (DLPFC). DLPFC is not only known to be involved in executive control functions but also known to be involved in cue reactivity to drugs. A specific disruption of functional connectivity between DLPFC and caudate has likewise been reported in heroin-addicted participants (Wang et al., 2013) which makes the neural correlates of pornography similar to those in drug addiction.

Another study that has investigated the structural neural correlates associated with hypersexuality used diffusion tensor imaging and reported higher mean diffusivity in a prefrontal white matter tract in a superior frontal region (Miner, Raymond, Mueller, Lloyd, & Lim, 2009) and a negative correlation between mean diffusivity in this tract and scores in a compulsive sexual behavior inventory. These authors likewise report more impulsive behavior in a Go-NoGo task in hypersexual compared with control participants.

Comparable inhibitory deficits have been demonstrated in cocaine-, MDMA-, methamphetamine-, tobacco-, and alcohol-dependent populations (Smith, Mattick, Jamadar, & Iredale, 2014).

Another study that investigated brain structure in hypersexuality by means of voxel-based morphometry might be of interest here, although the sample consisted of frontotemporal dementia patients (Perry et al., 2014). The authors report an association between right ventral putamen and pallidum atrophy and reward-seeking behavior. However, the authors correlated gray matter with a reward-seeking score that included other behavioral variants such as overeating (78%), increased alcohol or drug use (26%), in addition to hypersexuality (17%).

To summarize, the neuroimaging evidence points at an involvement of brain areas related to reward processing, including the nucleus accumbens (or more generally the striatum) and the VTA, prefrontal structures as well as limbic structures such as the amygdala and the hypothalamus in sexual arousal and potentially also hypersexuality.

5. LESION EVIDENCE OF HYPERSEXUALITY

Naturally occurring or therapeutic brain lesions have resulted in behavior that might be termed hypersexual. Since some of the evidence consists of single cases only, the results should be treated with caution. However, at the current stage of research, where comprehensive studies investigating the neurobiology of hypersexuality are sparse, they might be informative. The areas of interest hypothesized as involved in hypersexuality from the perspective of lesion studies include frontal and temporal lobes and hypothalamus.

In a single case report on a 25-year-old patient suffering from psychosis and hypersexuality, the patient was reported to have a frontal lesion secondary to neuroborreliosis (Stein, Solvason, Biggart, & Spiegel, 1996). In a 47-year-old man with a history of obsessive–compulsive disorder who showed signs of hypersexuality, a single-photon emission computerized tomography scan revealed lower perfusion in both temporal lobes, frontal cortex, and the ACC (Stein, Hugo, Oosthuizen, Hawkridge, & van Heerden, 2000). Furthermore, blood flow in basal ganglia and thalamus was asymmetric with decreased flow in the right hemisphere.

More evidence for the involvement of the temporal lobes in hypersexuality comes from bilateral lesions in the temporal lobes that have been shown to result in the Klüver–Bucy syndrome first described in 1939

(Klüver & Bucy, 1997) characterized by hypersexuality and other social behavioral disturbances (Wood, 1958). Originally, Klüver and Bucy surgically removed the temporal lobes including the amygdala in rhesus monkeys and observed a phenomenon they termed "Seelenblindheit" (psychic blindness). Monkeys were observed while handling a snake without showing any fear, showed strong tendencies to put objects into the mouth (oral tendencies), and to react strongly to visual stimuli. Moreover, changes in emotional and sexual behavior were observed (eg, attempts to mate with other species and objects). The Klüver–Bucy syndrome was also observed in bilateral temporal lesions in humans manifesting as hypersexuality, bulimia, and placidity (Góscínski, Kwiatkowski, Polak, Orlowiejska, & Partyk, 1997). Komisaruk and colleagues mentioned the hypothesis that surgical removal of the temporal lobe may lead to an inability to discriminate appropriate sexual objects, while it may at the same time lead to a reduction in social inhibition and an increase in sexual desire (Komisaruk & Rodriguez Del Cerro, 2015).

Likewise tumors in the temporal lobe (Blustein & Seeman, 1972) as well as temporal lobe strokes have been reported to result in hypersexuality (Monga, Monga, Raina, & Hardjasudarma, 1986). A single case of a 75-year-old man who underwent neurosurgery because of hydrocephalus resulting in a shunt in the septum reports that the man started approaching female patients inappropriately (Gorman & Cummings, 1992).

Two other single cases report lesions in the hypothalamus leading to hypersexual behavior. One described an infarct in the right thalamus and hypothalamus leading to hypomania and hypersexuality; the other study reported a left midbrain–hypothalamic glioma accompanied by pedophelia and hypersexuality (Miller, Cummings, McIntyre, Ebers, & Grode, 1986). Interestingly, in the 1970s therapeutic brain surgery was performed on the hypothalamus in an attempt to treat pedophelia and other sexual delinquencies (Dieckmann, Schneider-Jonietz, & Schneider, 1988).

To summarize, the evidence from lesion studies points at an involvement of frontal and temporal lobe as well as hypothalamus and the septum. The prevailing view is that frontal lobe lesions may result in disinhibition, whereas temporal lobe lesions can result in higher sexual drive.

6. EVIDENCE FROM OTHER NEUROLOGICAL DISEASES ACCOMPANIED BY HYPERSEXUALITY

In line with the previously discussed studies on brain lesion studies that reported hypersexual behavior, multiple sclerosis patients with frontal and periventricular lesions have been observed to show signs of disinhibition and hypersexuality (Gondim & Thomas, 2001; Huws, Shubsachs, & Taylor, 1991). Similarly, hypersexuality and disinhibition have been reported in the context of dementia (Cipriani, Ulivi, Danti, Lucetti, & Nuti, 2015), potentially caused by atrophy in frontal and temporal cortices.

Beyond diseases affecting frontal and temporal lobes, hypersexuality is likewise often observed in diseases that affect the striatum. Hypersexuality is frequently observed in Huntington's disease (Janati, 1985; Jhanjee, Anand, & Bajaj, 2011) as well as in Parkinson's disease patients who receive L-dopa therapy (Kenangil, Ozekmekçi, Sohtaoglu, & Erginöz, 2010). It has been reported that Parkinson's patients who receive dopamine agonist therapy have a 3.5% higher likelihood to be affected by hypersexuality. A more recent study estimates a higher prevalence of about 7% of hypersexuality in Parkinson's disease or its therapy (Hassan et al., 2011). Also animal studies in monkeys have shown that the interaction of dopamine drugs and sexual cues can enhance sexual activity (Pomerantz, 1990). Interestingly, not only dopaminergic pharmacotherapy but also deep brain stimulation in the subthalamic nucleus in Parkinson's patients has been shown to elicit hypersexuality (Romito et al., 2002).

Neuroimaging studies in Parkinson's patients with hypersexuality point toward a strong involvement of the striatum and the frontal cortex. It has been shown that greater brain activation in response to sexual stimuli in the striatum, ACC, and orbitofrontal cortex was associated with enhanced sexual desire in these patients (Politis et al., 2013). However, when patients were off L-dopa medication, the fMRI data showed decreases in activation in these areas. The authors interpret this pattern of responses as evidence that dopaminergic drugs release the brain from inhibition thereby contributing to compulsive sexual behavior (Weintraub et al., 2010). Similarly a positron emission tomography study revealed stronger striatal dopamine release in Parkinson's patients with impulse control disorders following reward cues compared to a control group of Parkinson's patients without impulse control disorders (O'Sullivan et al., 2011).

Epilepsy has also been associated with hypersexual behavior (Rees, Fowler, & Maas, 2007). Seizures arising from fronto-limbic or more frequently from temporo-limbic circuits can lead to genital automatism and sexual gestures (Dobesberger et al., 2004). Seizures can also lead to ictal orgasms, which can be eliminated by lobectomy of the temporal lobe and removal of the hippocampus and the amygdala (Baird, Wilson, Bladin, Saling, & Reutens, 2004). Interestingly, these sexual ictal events have been more strongly reported for right-sided temporal foci than for left-sided ones, whereas sexual automatisms are more frequently seen in frontal seizures (Cummings, 1997). Epileptic patients (64%) were reported to have changes in sexual function after temporal lobe resection. Improved sexuality was more frequently reported than unwelcomed decreases (Baird, Wilson, Bladin, Saling, & Reutens, 2003). A report from the 1970s mentioned patients with temporal lobe epilepsy were characterized as hyposexual before surgery, but became hypersexual after unilateral lobectomy that most likely involved hippocampus and amygdala in one hemisphere (Blumer, 1970). Interestingly, in the two patients who experienced seizures again after the lobectomy, hypersexuality vanished.

The presented evidence from neurological diseases that are sometimes accompanied by hypersexuality also seems to point at an involvement of temporal lobes (in particular hippocampus and amygdala), frontal lobe, and striatum.

7. NEUROPHARMACOLOGY OF HYPERSEXUALITY

There is evidence that hypersexuality may be promoted by decreases in serotonin and increases in dopamine levels (Guarraci & Bolton, 2014). Drugs such as amphetamines and cocaine are known to increase sexual desire (Angrist & Gershon, 1976). As a consequence, serotonin reuptake inhibitors (to increase serotonin), as well as dopamine blockers have been suggested to be of use in the neuropharmacological treatment of hypersexuality. In a double-blind placebo controlled study, citalopram, a SSRI, has been shown to reduce frequency of masturbation, sexual drive, and pornography use in homosexual men showing compulsive sexual behavior (Wainberg et al., 2006). Similarly Fluoxetine has been shown to reduce hypersexuality and paraphilias in men (Kafka & Prentky, 1992).

Antiandrogen medications such as cyproterone acetate (CPA) and medroxyprogesterone acetate (MPA) have been shown to be successful in decreasing the frequency and intensity of sexual desire as well as decreasing subjective sexual arousal (Krueger & Kaplan, 2002). The mechanism of action of CPA consists if it is binding to androgen receptors and thereby blocking testosterone uptake. MPA, on the other hand, acts as a progesterone and exerts negative feedback on the hypothalamic–pituitary axis; it accelerates testosterone metabolism and clearance; MPA may also bind to androgen receptors. However, antiandrogens have a high rate of negative side effects (Turner, Schöttle, Bradford, & Briken, 2014).

Taken together, the effectiveness of the different type of drugs points at an involvement of high dopamine, low serotonin, and high testosterone levels in the emergence of hypersexuality.

8. ANIMAL STUDIES ON HYPERSEXUALITY

Rats that have been lesioned in the limbic system, in particular in the septal region, have been shown to display increased sexual behavior (Rasmussen, Kaada, & Bruland, 1960). Similar effects have been observed after lesions in the mammillary region (Lisk, 1966). By contrast, direct stimulation of the limbic system in nonhuman primates has been shown to result in erections (MacLean, Denniston, & Dua, 1963). In line with the previously suggested association between frontal lesions and hypersexuality, lesions in the medial prefrontal cortex in male rats have been shown to result in disinhibited sexual behavior (Davis et al., 2010). In accordance with the above-mentioned connection between hypersexuality and the dopaminergic system, repeated methamphetamine exposure in male rats has been shown to result in compulsive sex-seeking behavior 2 weeks after the last administration (Frohmader, Lehman, Laviolette, & Coolen, 2011).

Interestingly, overproduction of ΔFosB, a protein that has been identified to play a crucial role in addiction and neural plasticity, has been shown to enhance sensitivity to sexual activity in Syrian hamsters (Hedges, Chakravarty, Nestler, & Meisel, 2009). It has also been demonstrated that sexual experiences increase ΔFosB concentrations in nucleus accumbens (Wallace et al., 2008). Further evidence for a link between substance addiction and sexual behavior has been suggested in a study in mice, where repeated sexual experiences lead to a higher sensitivity to amphetamines (Pitchers et al., 2010).

The animal studies underline the findings previously discussed in humans suggesting an involvement of frontal, temporal, and striatal brain regions in hypersexuality, and at the same time, stress the potential link to drug addiction.

9. GENETICS OF HYPERSEXUALITY

Initial evidence indicates that hypersexuality may be genetically determined, because patients have a high likelihood to have a parent with a similar condition (36%) (Schneider & Schneider, 1996). Many hypersexual individuals report having at least one family member with an addiction disorder

(81%). In line with previously reported evidence of a potential association between the dopaminergic system and hypersexuality, associations between genetic variants of the D1, D2, and D4 dopamine receptor (DRD1, DRD2, and DRD4) and age at first sexual intercourse was observed (Miller et al., 1999). Individuals with at least one 7-repeat allele in the DRD4 gene show a higher rate of promiscuous behavior (eg, having one night stands) and report more instances of sexual infidelity (Garcia et al., 2010). Individuals with a particular DRD2 genotype show a higher rate of sexual intercourse without use of contraceptives (Daw & Guo, 2011). The dopamine transporter gene (DAT1) seems to be predictive of the number of sexual partners and criminal conduct in men (Beaver, Wright, & Walsh, 2008). A very interesting evolutionary hypothesis has been suggested by Comings (1996). He reports data that individuals prone to addiction have offspring earlier, which at the same time impacts selection of genes associated with addiction. If, for example, individuals with addiction related genetic variants have children 5 years earlier than individuals without these genetic variants, the addiction alleles will reproduce faster, providing a selection advantage across generations.

10. CONCLUSION

Although research on the neurobiological underpinnings of hypersexuality is still rare, there is a considerable degree of concordance between brain regions implicated in excessive sexual behavior in neuroimaging and lesion studies as well as evidence from other neurological disorders that are frequently associated with hypersexuality and animal studies. The data seem to imply that alterations in frontal lobe, temporal lobe, in particular the amygdala and hippocampus, hypothalamus, septum, and reward-associated brain regions (eg, striatum, nucleus accumbens, VTA), play a prominent role in the emergence of hypersexuality. The sex hormone testosterone may be involved and genetic studies and neuropharmacology implicate involvement of the dopaminergic system. For now, it is unclear which brain regions elicit only disinhibition and thereby indirectly contribute to a higher rate of expression of sexuality and which areas are directly associated with an increase in sexual drive, since both phenomena may ultimately lead to increases in sexual behavior. In order to reach unequivocal conclusions on the role of the different brain regions, more research is needed.

In conclusion, we consider it important to reflect whether hypersexuality should be treated as a disorder (Frascella et al., 2010). Behavioral addictions and in particular hypersexuality should remind us of the fact that addictive behavior actually relies on our natural survival system. Sex is an essential component in survival of species since it is the pathway for reproduction. Therefore it is extremely important that sex is considered pleasurable and has primal rewarding properties, and although it may turn into an addiction at which point sex may be pursued in a dangerous and counterproductive way, the neural basis for addiction might actually serve very important purposes in primal goal pursuit of individuals.

REFERENCES

Angrist, B., & Gershon, S. (1976). Clinical effects of amphetamine and L-DOPA on sexuality and aggression. *Comprehensive Psychiatry, 17*(6), 715–722.

Baird, A. D., Wilson, S. J., Bladin, P. F., Saling, M. M., & Reutens, D. C. (2003). Sexual outcome after epilepsy surgery. *Epilepsy & Behavior, 4*(3), 268–278. http://doi.org/10.1016/S1525-5050(03)00085-4.

Baird, A. D., Wilson, S. J., Bladin, P. F., Saling, M. M., & Reutens, D. C. (2004). The amygdala and sexual drive: Insights from temporal lobe epilepsy surgery. *Annals of Neurology, 55*(1), 87–96. http://doi.org/10.1002/ana.10997.

Barth, R. J., & Kinder, B. N. (1987). The mislabeling of sexual impulsivity. *Journal of Sex & Marital Therapy, 13*(1), 15–23. http://doi.org/10.1080/00926238708403875.

Beaver, K. M., Wright, J. P., & Walsh, A. (2008). A gene-based evolutionary explanation for the association between criminal involvement and number of sex partners. *Biodemography and Social Biology, 54*(1), 47–55. http://doi.org/10.1080/19485565.2008.9989131.

Black, D. W., Kehrberg, L., Flumerfelt, D. L., & Schlosser, S. S. (1997). Characteristics of 36 subjects reporting compulsive sexual behavior. *The American Journal of Psychiatry, 154*, 243–249.

Blumer, D. (1970). Hypersexual episodes in temporal lobe epilepsy. *The American Journal of Psychiatry, 126*(8), 1099–1106.

Blustein, J., & Seeman, M. V. (1972). Brain tumors presenting as functional psychiatric disturbances. *Canadian Psychiatric Association Journal, 17*(2 Suppl. 2), SS59–SS63.

Carpenter, B. N., Reid, R. C., Garos, S., & Najavits, L. M. (2013). Personality disorder comorbidity in treatment-seeking men with hypersexual disorder. *Sexual Addiction & Compulsivity, 20*, 79–90.

Childress, A. R., Ehrman, R. N., Wang, Z., Li, Y., Sciortino, N., Hakun, J., et al. (2008). Prelude to passion: Limbic activation by "unseen" drug and sexual cues. *PLoS One, 3*(1), e1506. http://doi.org/10.1371/journal.pone.0001506.

Cipriani, G., Ulivi, M., Danti, S., Lucetti, C., & Nuti, A. (2015). Sexual disinhibition and dementia. *Psychogeriatrics, 16*, 145–153. http://doi.org/10.1111/psyg.12143.

Comings, D. E. (1996). *The gene bomb: Does higher education and advanced technology accelerate the selection of genes for learning disorders, ADHD, addictive, and disruptive behaviors?* Duarte, CA: Hope Press. 304 pp.

Cummings, J. L. (1997). Neuropsychiatric manifestations of right hemisphere lesions. *Brain and Language, 57*(1), 22–37. http://doi.org/10.1006/brln.1997.1832.

Davis, J. F., Loos, M., Di Sebastiano, A. R., Brown, J. L., Lehman, M. N., & Coolen, L. M. (2010). Lesions of the medial prefrontal cortex cause maladaptive sexual behavior in male rats. *Biological Psychiatry*, *67*(12), 1199–1204.

Daw, J., & Guo, G. (2011). The influence of three genes on whether adolescents use contraception, USA 1994–2002. *Population Studies*, *65*(3), 253–271. http://doi.org/10.1080/00324728.2011.598942.

Dieckmann, G., Schneider-Jonietz, B., & Schneider, H. (1988). Psychiatric and neuropsychological findings after stereotactic hypothalamotomy, in cases of extreme sexual aggressivity. *Acta Neurochirurgica. Supplementum*, *44*, 163–166.

Dobesberger, J., Walser, G., Unterberger, I., Embacher, N., Luef, G., Bauer, G., et al. (2004). Genital automatisms: A video-EEG study in patients with medically refractory seizures. *Epilepsia*, *45*(7), 777–780. http://doi.org/10.1111/j.0013-9580.2004.44003.x.

Frascella, J., Potenza, M. N., Brown, L. L., & Childress, A. R. (2010). Shared brain vulnerabilities open the way for nonsubstance addictions: Carving addiction at a new joint? *Annals of the New York Academy of Sciences*, *1187*, 294–315. http://doi.org/10.1111/j.1749-6632.2009.05420.x.

Frohmader, K. S., Lehman, M. N., Laviolette, S. R., & Coolen, L. M. (2011). Concurrent exposure to methamphetamine and sexual behavior enhances subsequent drug reward and causes compulsive sexual behavior in male rats. *Journal of Neuroscience*, *31*(45), 16473–16482. http://doi.org/10.1523/JNEUROSCI.4013-11.2011.

Garcia, J. R., MacKillop, J., Aller, E. L., Merriwether, A. M., Wilson, D. S., & Lum, J. K. (2010). Associations between dopamine D4 receptor gene variation with both infidelity and sexual promiscuity. *PLoS One*, *5*(11), e14162. http://doi.org/10.1371/journal.pone.0014162.

Garcia, F. D., & Thibaut, F. (2010). Sexual addictions. *The American Journal of Drug and Alcohol Abuse*, *36*(5), 254–260. http://doi.org/10.3109/00952990.2010.503823.

Gondim, F. A., & Thomas, F. P. (2001). Episodic hyperlibidinism in multiple sclerosis. *Multiple Sclerosis*, 7(1), 67–70.

Gorman, D. G., & Cummings, J. L. (1992). Hypersexuality following septal injury. *Archives of Neurology*, *49*(3), 308–310.

Góscínski, I., Kwiatkowski, S., Polak, J., Orlowiejska, M., & Partyk, A. (1997). The Kluver-Bucy syndrome. *Journal of Neurosurgical Sciences*, *41*(3), 269–272.

Guarraci, F. A., & Bolton, J. L. (2014). "Sexy stimulants": The interaction between psychomotor stimulants and sexual behavior in the female brain. *Pharmacology, Biochemistry, and Behavior*, *121*, 53–61. http://doi.org/10.1016/j.pbb.2013.11.006.

Hassan, A., Bower, J. H., Kumar, N., Matsumoto, J. Y., Fealey, R. D., Josephs, K. A., et al. (2011). Dopamine agonist-triggered pathological behaviors: Surveillance in the PD clinic reveals high frequencies. *Parkinsonism & Related Disorders*, *17*(4), 260–264. http://doi.org/10.1016/j.parkreldis.2011.01.009.

Hedges, V. L., Chakravarty, S., Nestler, E. J., & Meisel, R. L. (2009). ΔFosB overexpression in the nucleus accumbens enhances sexual reward in female Syrian hamsters. *Genes, Brain, and Behavior*, *8*(4), 442–449. http://doi.org/10.1111/j.1601-183X.2009.00491.x.

Holstege, G., Georgiadis, J. R., Paans, A. M. J., Meiners, L. C., van der Graaf, F. H. C. E., & Reinders, A. A. T. S. (2003). Brain activation during human male ejaculation. *The Journal of Neuroscience*, *23*, 9185–9193.

Huws, R., Shubsachs, A. P., & Taylor, P. J. (1991). Hypersexuality, fetishism and multiple sclerosis. *British Journal of Psychiatry*, *158*, 280–281.

Janati, A. (1985). Kluver-Bucy syndrome in Huntington's chorea. *The Journal of Nervous and Mental Disease*, *173*(10), 632–635.

Jhanjee, A., Anand, K. S., & Bajaj, B. K. (2011). Hypersexual features in Huntington's disease. *Singapore Medical Journal*, *52*(6), e131–e133.

Jia, Z.-J., Yan, S.-Y., Bao, Y.-P., Lian, Z., Zhang, H.-R., & Liu, Z.-M. (2013). Sexual behavior differences between amphetamine-type stimulants users and heroin users. *Journal of Addiction Medicine*, 7(6), 422–427. http://doi.org/10.1097/ADM.0b013e3182a952b2.

Kafka, M. P. (1997). Hypersexual desire in males: An operational definition and clinical implications for males with paraphilias and paraphilia-related disorders. *Archives of Sexual Behavior, 26*(5), 505–526. http://doi.org/10.1023/A:1024507922470.

Kafka, M. P., & Hennen, J. (2002). A DSM-IV axis I comorbidity study of males ($n = 120$) with paraphilias and paraphilia-related disorders. *Sexual Abuse: A Journal of Research and Treatment, 14*(4), 349–366. http://doi.org/10.1023/A:1020007004436.

Kafka, M. P., & Hennen, J. (2003). Hypersexual desire in males: Are males with paraphilias different from males with paraphilia-related disorders? *Sexual Abuse: A Journal of Research and Treatment, 15*(4), 307–321. http://doi.org/10.1023/A:1025000227956.

Kafka, M. P., & Prentky, R. (1992). Fluoxetine treatment of nonparaphilic sexual addictions and paraphilias in men. *Journal of Clinical Psychiatry, 53*, 351–358.

Kenangil, G., Ozekmekçi, S., Sohtaoglu, M., & Erginöz, E. (2010). Compulsive behaviors in patients with Parkinson's disease. *The Neurologist, 16*(3), 192–195. http://doi.org/10.1097/NRL.0b013e31819f952b.

Kingston, D. A., & Firestone, P. (2008). Problematic hypersexuality: A review of conceptualization and diagnosis. *Sexual Addiction & Compulsivity, 15*(4), 284–310. http://doi.org/10.1080/10720160802289249.

Kinsey, A. C., Pomeroy, W. B., & Martin, C. E. (1948). *Sexual behavior in the human male,* (pp. 804). Philadelphia: W. B. Saunders.

Klüver, H., & Bucy, P. C. (1997). Preliminary analysis of functions of the temporal lobes in monkeys. 1939. *The Journal of Neuropsychiatry and Clinical Neurosciences, 9*, 606–620.

Komisaruk, B. R., & Rodriguez Del Cerro, M. C. (2015). Human sexual behavior related to pathology and activity of the brain. *Handbook of Clinical Neurology, 130*, 109–119. http://doi.org/10.1016/B978-0-444-63247-0.00006-7.

Komisaruk, B. R., & Whipple, B. (2005). Functional MRI of the brain during orgasm in women. *Annual Review of Sex Research, 16*, 62–86.

Komisaruk, B. R., Whipple, B., Crawford, A., Grimes, S., Liu, W.-C., Kalnin, A., et al. (2004). Brain activation during vaginocervical self-stimulation and orgasm in women with complete spinal cord injury: fMRI evidence of mediation by the vagus nerves. *Brain Research, 1024*(1–2), 77–88.

Komisaruk, B. R., Wise, N., Frangos, E., Birbano, W., & Allen, K. (2011). *An fMRI video animation time-course analysis of brain regions activated during self-stimulation to orgasm in women.* Poster No. 495.03/SS27. Neuroscience Meeting Planner. Washington, DC: Society for Neuroscience, Online.

Krueger, R. B., & Kaplan, M. S. (2002). Behavioral and psychopharmacological treatment of the paraphilic and hypersexual disorders. *Journal of Psychiatric Practice, 8*(1), 21.

Kühn, S., & Gallinat, J. (2011a). A quantitative meta-analysis on cue-induced male sexual arousal. *The Journal of Sexual Medicine, 8*(8), 2269–2275. http://doi.org/10.1111/j.1743-6109.2011.02322.x.

Kühn, S., & Gallinat, J. (2011b). Common biology of craving across legal and illegal drugs—A quantitative meta-analysis of cue-reactivity brain response. *European Journal of Neuroscience, 33*, 1318–1326.

Kühn, S., & Gallinat, J. (2014). Brain structure and functional connectivity associated with pornography consumption: The brain on porn. *JAMA Psychiatry, 71*, 827–834. http://doi.org/10.1001/jamapsychiatry.2014.93.

Kuzma, J. M., & Black, D. W. (2008). Epidemiology, prevalence, and natural history of compulsive sexual behavior. *Psychiatric Clinics of North America, 31*, 603–611.

Lisk, R. D. (1966). Increased sexual behavior in the male rat following lesions in the mammillary region. *Journal of Experimental Zoology, 161*(1), 129–136. http://doi.org/10.1002/jez.1401610112.
Love, T., Laier, C., Brand, M., Hatch, L., & Hajela, R. (2015). Neuroscience of internet pornography addiction: A review and update. *Behavioral Sciences (Basel, Switzerland), 5*(3), 388–433. http://doi.org/10.3390/bs5030388.
MacLean, P. D., Denniston, R. H., & Dua, S. (1963). Further studies on cerebral representation of penile erection: Caudal thalamus, midbrain, and pons. *Journal of Neurophysiology, 26*(2), 273–293.
Mick, T. M., & Hollander, E. (2006). Impulsive-compulsive sexual behavior. *CNS Spectrums, 11*(12), 944–955. http://doi.org/10.1017/S1092852900015133.
Miller, B. L., Cummings, J. L., McIntyre, H., Ebers, G., & Grode, M. (1986). Hypersexuality or altered sexual preference following brain injury. *Journal of Neurology, Neurosurgery, and Psychiatry, 49*(8), 867–873.
Miller, W. B., Pasta, D. J., MacMurray, J., Chiu, C., Wu, H., & Comings, D. E. (1999). Dopamine receptor genes are associated with age at first sexual intercourse. *Journal of Biosocial Science, 31*(1), 43–54.
Miner, M. H., Raymond, N., Mueller, B. A., Lloyd, M., & Lim, K. O. (2009). Preliminary investigation of the impulsive and neuroanatomical characteristics of compulsive sexual behavior. *Psychiatry Research, 174*(2), 146–151. http://doi.org/10.1016/j.pscychresns.2009.04.008.
Monga, T. N., Monga, M., Raina, M. S., & Hardjasudarma, M. (1986). Hypersexuality in stroke. *Archives of Physical Medicine and Rehabilitation, 67*(6), 415–417.
O'Sullivan, S. S., Wu, K., Politis, M., Lawrence, A. D., Evans, A. H., Bose, S. K., et al. (2011). Cue-induced striatal dopamine release in Parkinson's disease-associated impulsive-compulsive behaviours. *Brain, 134*(4), 969–978. http://doi.org/10.1093/brain/awr003.
Perry, D. C., Sturm, V. E., Seeley, W. W., Miller, B. L., Kramer, J. H., & Rosen, H. J. (2014). Anatomical correlates of reward-seeking behaviours in behavioural variant frontotemporal dementia. *Brain, 137*(Pt. 6), 1621–1626. http://doi.org/10.1093/brain/awu075.
Pitchers, K. K., Pitchers, K. K., Balfour, M. E., Balfour, M. E., Lehman, M. N., Lehman, M. N., et al. (2010). Neuroplasticity in the mesolimbic system induced by natural reward and subsequent reward abstinence. *Biological Psychiatry, 67*(9), 872–879. http://doi.org/10.1016/j.biopsych.2009.09.036.
Politis, M., Loane, C., Wu, K., O'Sullivan, S. S., Woodhead, Z., Kiferle, L., et al. (2013). Neural response to visual sexual cues in dopamine treatment-linked hypersexuality in Parkinson's disease. *Brain, 136*(Pt. 2), 400–411. http://doi.org/10.1093/brain/aws326.
Pomerantz, S. M. (1990). Apomorphine facilitates male sexual behavior of rhesus monkeys. *Pharmacology, Biochemistry, and Behavior, 35*(3), 659–664.
Rasmussen, E. W., Kaada, B. R., & Bruland, H. (1960). Effects of neocortical and limbic lesions on the sex drive in rats. *Acta Physiologica Scandinavica, 50*, 126–127.
Raymond, N. C., Coleman, E., & Miner, M. H. (2003). Psychiatric comorbidity and compulsive/impulsive traits in compulsive sexual behavior. *Comprehensive Psychiatry, 44*, 370–380.
Rees, P. M., Fowler, C. J., & Maas, C. P. (2007). Sexual function in men and women with neurological disorders. *Lancet, 369*(9560), 512–525. http://doi.org/10.1016/S0140-6736(07)60238-4.
Reid, R. C., & Kafka, M. P. (2014). Controversies about hypersexual disorder and the DSM-5. *Current Sexual Health Reports, 6*(4), 259–264. http://doi.org/10.1007/s11930-014-0031-9.
Robinson, T. E., & Berridge, K. C. (2008). The incentive sensitization theory of addiction: Some current issues. *Philosophical Transactions: Biological Sciences, 363*(1507), 3137–3146. http://doi.org/10.2307/20208728?ref=search-gateway:3ba4ea4013023e57c72edd57a8ed25f8.

Romito, L. M., Raja, M., Daniele, A., Contarino, M. F., Bentivoglio, A. R., Barbier, A., et al. (2002). Transient mania with hypersexuality after surgery for high frequency stimulation of the subthalamic nucleus in Parkinson's disease. *Movement Disorders: Official Journal of the Movement Disorder Society, 17*(6), 1371–1374. http://doi.org/10.1002/mds.10265.
Schneider, J. P., & Schneider, B. H. (1996). Couple recovery from sexual addiction/co addiction: Results of a survey of 88 marriages. *Sexual Addiction & Compulsivity, 3*(2), 111–126. http://doi.org/10.1080/10720169608400106.
Smith, J. L., Mattick, R. P., Jamadar, S. D., & Iredale, J. M. (2014). Deficits in behavioural inhibition in substance abuse and addiction: A meta-analysis. *Drug and Alcohol Dependence, 145*, 1–33. http://doi.org/10.1016/j.drugalcdep.2014.08.009.
Spauwen, L. W. L., Niekamp, A. M., Hoebe, C. J. P. A., & Dukers-Muijrers, N. H. T. M. (2015). Drug use, sexual risk behaviour and sexually transmitted infections among swingers: A cross-sectional study in the Netherlands. *Sexually Transmitted Infections, 91*(1), 31–36. http://doi.org/10.1136/sextrans-2014-051626.
Steele, V. R., Staley, C., Fong, T., & Prause, N. (2013). Sexual desire, not hypersexuality, is related to neurophysiological responses elicited by sexual images. *Socioaffective Neuroscience & Psychology, 3*, 20770. http://doi.org/10.3402/snp.v3i0.20770.
Stein, D. J., Hugo, F., Oosthuizen, P., Hawkridge, S. M., & van Heerden, B. (2000). Neuropsychiatry of hypersexuality. *CNS Spectrums, 5*(1), 36–46.
Stein, S. L., Solvason, H. B., Biggart, E., & Spiegel, D. (1996). A 25-year-old woman with hallucinations, hypersexuality, nightmares, and a rash. *The American Journal of Psychiatry, 153*, 545–551.
Turner, D., Schöttle, D., Bradford, J., & Briken, P. (2014). Assessment methods and management of hypersexuality and paraphilic disorders. *Current Opinion in Psychiatry, 27*(6), 413–422. http://doi.org/10.1097/YCO.0000000000000099.
Voon, V., Mole, T. B., Banca, P., Porter, L., Morris, L., Mitchell, S., et al. (2014). Neural correlates of sexual cue reactivity in individuals with and without compulsive sexual behaviours. *PLoS One, 9*(7), e102419. http://doi.org/10.1371/journal.pone.0102419.
Wainberg, M. L., Muench, F., Morgenstern, J., Hollander, E., Irwin, T. W., Parsons, J. T., et al. (2006). A double-blind study of citalopram versus placebo in the treatment of compulsive sexual behaviors in gay and bisexual men. *The Journal of Clinical Psychiatry, 67*(12), 1968–1973.
Wallace, D. L., Vialou, V., Rios, L., Carle-Florence, T. L., Chakravarty, S., Kumar, A., et al. (2008). The influence of FosB in the nucleus accumbens on natural reward-related behavior. *Journal of Neuroscience, 28*(41), 10272–10277. http://doi.org/10.1523/JNEUROSCI.1531-08.2008.
Wang, Y., Zhu, J., Li, Q., Li, W., Wu, N., Zheng, Y., et al. (2013). Altered fronto-striatal and fronto-cerebellar circuits in heroin-dependent individuals: A resting-state FMRI study. *PLoS One, 8*(3), e58098. http://doi.org/10.1371/journal.pone.0058098.
Watts, C., & Hilton, D. (2011). Pornography addiction: A neuroscience perspective. *Surgical Neurology International, 2*(1), 19. http://doi.org/10.4103/2152-7806.76977.
Weintraub, D., Koester, J., Potenza, M. N., Siderowf, A. D., Stacy, M., Voon, V., et al. (2010). Impulse control disorders in Parkinson disease: A cross-sectional study of 3090 patients. *Archives of Neurology, 67*(5), 589–595. http://doi.org/10.1001/archneurol.2010.65.
Wood, C. D. (1958). Behavioral changes following discrete lesions of temporal lobe structures. *Neurology, 8*(3), 215–220.

CHAPTER FOUR

Psychological and Neurobiological Correlates of Food Addiction

E. Kalon[*,†,1], J.Y. Hong[†], C. Tobin[*,‡], T. Schulte[*,†]
[*]Palo Alto University, Palo Alto, CA, United States
[†]SRI International, Menlo Park, CA, United States
[‡]National Center for PTSD, VA Palo Alto Health Care System Menlo Park Division, Menlo Park, CA, United States
[1]Corresponding author: e-mail address: ekalon@paloaltou.edu

Contents

Abstract

Food addiction (FA) is loosely defined as hedonic eating behavior involving the consumption of highly palatable foods (ie, foods high in salt, fat, and sugar) in quantities beyond homeostatic energy requirements. FA shares some common symptomology with other pathological eating disorders, such as binge eating. Current theories suggest that FA shares both behavioral similarities and overlapping neural correlates to other substance addictions. Although preliminary, neuroimaging studies in response to food cues and the consumption of highly palatable food in individuals with FA compared to healthy controls have shown differing activation patterns and connectivity in brain reward circuits including regions such as the striatum, amygdala, orbitofrontal cortex,

International Review of Neurobiology, Volume 129
ISSN 0074-7742
http://dx.doi.org/10.1016/bs.irn.2016.06.003

insula, and nucleus accumbens. Additional effects have been noted in the hypothalamus, a brain area responsible for regulating eating behaviors and peripheral satiety networks. FA is highly impacted by impulsivity and mood. Chronic stress can negatively affect hypothalamic–pituitary–adrenal axis functioning, thus influencing eating behavior and increasing desirability of highly palatable foods. Future work will require clearly defining FA as a distinct diagnosis from other eating disorders.

1. INTRODUCTION

The primary focus of this chapter is to discuss the current understanding of food addiction (FA) in light of neurobehavioral models based on findings from advanced neuroimaging tools. Recent literature suggests that biological, psychological, behavioral, and nutritional components play a part in the etiology and persistence of FA (Gearhardt et al., 2011; Parylak, Koob, & Zorrilla, 2011; Singh, 2014; Sinha & Jastreboff, 2013; Ziauddeen, Alonso-Alonso, Hill, Kelley, & Khan, 2015). In the United States, more than two-thirds of adults are considered overweight or obese, and obesity is linked to an array of health risks, ranging from type 2 diabetes and heart disease to breast, colon, endometrial, and kidney cancer (The National Institute of Diabetes and Digestive and Kidney Diseases, 2012). Although "food addiction" and "obesity" are often used interchangeably, these designations correspond to unique underlying concepts. FA is loosely defined as a behavior involving the uncontrollable urge or insatiable desire to continue eating past what would be considered a physical or metabolic need (Parylak et al., 2011) whereas obesity is defined by a body mass index (BMI) of 30 and above (National Institutes of Health & Department of Health and Human Services, n.d.). A person can have a FA and not be obese. Conversely, one can be obese and not have a FA, although obesity may be a consequence of FA, and therefore FA incidence may be higher among this population (Meule, 2011; Pursey, Stanwell, Gearhardt, Collins, & Burrows, 2014).

From a theoretical and research-based viewpoint, it is important to distinguish between FA and other eating disorders. *The Diagnostic and Statistical Manual, 5th Edition* (DSM-5) describes criteria for "Feeding and Eating Disorders" (American Psychiatric Association, 2013a) of which the three most prevalent are anorexia nervosa, bulimia nervosa, and binge-eating disorder. Anorexia nervosa is characterized by restriction of energy intake relative to requirements and significantly low body weight. Bulimia nervosa includes episodes of binge-eating and compensatory behaviors to prevent weight gain. Lastly, binge-eating disorder involves recurrent binge-eating episodes along with extreme distress surrounding the binge-eating behavior (American Psychiatric Association, 2013a). Community studies including participants with a diverse weight range showed that individuals with FA, but not binge-eating disorder, report significant levels of impairment and distress, including depressive symptoms, impulsivity, and negative affect (Gearhardt, Boswell, & White, 2014). Among individuals who meet criteria for FA, the frequency of binge-eating disorder ranges from 27% to 30%, suggesting a high comorbidity between the two conditions (Davis et al., 2011; Gearhardt, Boswell, & White, 2014). While there is a strong association between FA and eating disorders, predominantly bulimia nervosa and binge-eating disorder, they have distinctly different presentations, particularly related to the frequency and level of symptomology. FA appears to be marked by more severe depression, negative affect, and general levels of distress compared to other eating disorders.

As a concept, addiction to food is complex, and its meaning has evolved over time. It is necessary to operationalize this notion in order to provide a framework for further investigation. In a review of over 40 papers on the definition of addiction, Sussman and Sussman (2011) formulated a list of criteria: (1) partaking in behavior due to appetitive effects; (2) spending a great deal of time thinking about, obtaining, using, and recovering from the effects of the substance; (3) satiation, described as a period of time directly after the use of a substance when the addictive behavior temporarily subsides only to return quite quickly as the effects dissipate; (4) impulsivity or loss of control over the behavior; and (5) suffering negative psychosocial, emotional, and health consequences. The concept of FA will be evaluated using these criteria. Addiction, as defined by Sussman and Sussman (2011), closely resembles the DSM-5 criteria for substance use disorders (American Psychiatric Association, 2013b). The Yale Food Addiction Scale Version 2.0 (YFAS 2.0), the only currently existing operational measure of FA, is based on DSM-5 criteria (Gearhardt, Corbin, & Brownell, 2016). The YFAS 2.0 maps onto the DSM-5 criteria for addiction by asking questions about time spent on eating and the quantity of food consumed, unsuccessful efforts to cut down despite high motivation, time spent on obtaining food, presence of cravings, eating habits negatively impacting obligations and social relations, eating despite negative physical consequences, a need for greater food intake to achieve satiety (ie, tolerance), and negative physiological or psychological feelings when eating certain foods is stopped (ie, withdrawal) (American Psychiatric Association, 2013b; Gearhardt et al., 2016).

A meta-analysis including 28 studies found a weighted mean prevalence for FA of 19.9% among adults in the United States (Pursey et al., 2014). When looking at studies that addressed sex differences specifically, rates were greater in woman than in men (12.2% vs 6.4%). Overweight/obese subjects had higher rates of FA than those with a healthy BMI (24.9% vs 11.1%). Lastly, FA also appears to be more prevalent in individuals 35 years and older than in individuals younger than 35 (22.2% vs 17.0%). Although these findings should be interpreted with caution, because the majority of participants were female and obese, they provide initial insight into the number of people in the United States with FA (Pursey et al., 2014).

Neuroimaging permits researchers to study the effects of food-related stimuli on specific brain regions and their intrinsic functional connectivity. Specifically, functional magnetic resonance imaging (fMRI) can be used to measure the blood oxygenation level-dependent response to stimuli or at rest. A variety of eating behaviors, including the processing of tastes, appearances, and scents of food, and satiety, reward, motivation, reappraisal, craving, and consumption associated with food have been investigated with fMRI (Giuliani & Pfeifer, 2015; Huerta, Sarkar, Duong, Laird, & Fox, 2014; Jiang, Soussignan, Schaal, & Royet, 2015; Murdaugh, Cox, Cook, & Weller, 2012; Robinson, Fischer, Ahuja, Lesser, & Maniates, 2016; Rolls, 2015; Rolls, Kellerhals, & Nichols, 2015; Simmons et al., 2014; Thomas et al., 2015; van Bloemendaal et al., 2015; Wang, Smith, & Delgado, 2016). Evaluation of FA has demonstrated alterations in brain regions involved in reward processing, homeostatic regulation, emotional reactivity, and executive control (Gearhardt, Boswell, & Potenza, 2014; Lao-Kaim et al., 2015; Simon et al., 2016; Ziauddeen, Farooqi, & Fletcher, 2012). Because neuroimaging of FA is still in preliminary stages, only a few studies are currently available to review.

2. FACTORS THAT LEAD TO THE FORMATION OF FA

2.1 Hyperpalatable Foods

Specific types of foods, frequently referred to as "palatable" or "hyperpalatable," due to their high content of salt, sugar, and fat (Gearhardt, Grilo, DiLeone, Brownell, & Potenza, 2011), are considered to have addictive potential (de Macedo, de Freitas, & da Silva Torres, 2016) because they contain a high density of nutrients or additives (Meule, 2015). Schulte, Avena, and Gearhardt (2015) asked a group of 120 undergraduate students to indicate which among a nutritionally varied list of 35 foods were most addictive. Analyses revealed that the most common foods chosen were processed, had a high-fat content, and a high glycemic load, a measure of the extent to which a carbohydrate affects blood sugar levels (Monro & Shaw, 2008). It is possible that diets high in palatable foods along with other risk factors can increase risk for developing a FA (Gearhardt, Davis, Kuschner, & Brownell, 2011). For example, it has been shown with fMRI that even in healthy young women, viewing pictures of highly palatable food or drinks activated brain regions of the reward circuitry (Gearhardt, Yokum, et al., 2011).

2.2 Operant Conditioning

Operant conditioning can help explain how an individual may transition from occasional, nonpathological consumption of hyperpalatable foods to problematic, addictive eating. The evolution of drug addiction may be explained by a learned process wherein a person is initially motivated by the rewarding aspects of a substance, such as feeling "high" or experiencing elevated mood (positive reinforcement) (Koob, 2000; Weiss et al., 2001). As time progresses, motivation shifts from desire for positive experiences to avoidance of aversive experiences, such as those that accompany withdrawal. This avoidance is achieved through continued use of the substance despite the loss of the original euphoric feeling (negative reinforcement) (Koob, 2000, 2003; Weiss et al., 2001). It has been hypothesized that this same model applies to hyperpalatable foods leading to FA (Meule & Kubler, 2012). Initially, one may be motivated to eat specific energy-dense foods due to the rewarding feelings elicited when eating such foods (Parylak et al., 2011). Over time, the consumption of highly palatable foods may lead to neuroadaptations in brain reward centers involving the downregulation of D2 receptors, as seen in other substance addictions: motivation switches to a desire to ameliorate negative emotional or physiological states, such as depression, anxiety, irritability, or other somatic symptoms related to absence of the highly palatable food (de Macedo et al., 2016; Meule & Kubler, 2012; Parylak et al., 2011). To date, most of the evidence for this type of neuroplasticity in FA comes from animal studies (Ahmed et al., 2014; Johnson & Kenny, 2010; van de Giessen et al., 2013).

2.3 Mood and Stress

There is evidence that those with FA or FA symptomology may be using addictive eating behaviors to cope with negative emotional states

(Micanti et al., 2016). For example, binge-eating behavior is associated with psychosocial factors such as negative affect and mood dysregulation (Micanti et al., 2016), weight cycling (Zwaan, Engeli, & Muller, 2015), body dissatisfaction (Goldschmidt, Wall, Choo, Becker, & Neumark-Sztainer, 2016), fear of self-compassion (Kelly, Vimalakanthan, & Carter, 2014), and neuroticism (Womble et al., 2001). Individuals who are underweight or normal weight report lower food consumption when experiencing negative emotions than when experiencing positive emotions. The inverse is true for overweight individuals, who consume more food when experiencing negative emotions (Geliebter & Aversa, 2003). Similar results were seen in a group of women who scored high on the YFAS and showed significantly higher levels of depression than those whose scores did not indicate FA (Berenson, Laz, Pohlmeier, Rahman, & Cunningham, 2015. There is also substantial evidence to support the connection between stress and addiction (Cui et al., 2013; Koob, 2013; Spanagel, Noori, & Heilig, 2014; Taylor et al., 2014). Stress has been found to be associated with a change in eating patterns, including binging episodes and craving highly palatable foods (Sinha & Jastreboff, 2013). Negative affect and stress may also represent withdrawal in individuals with FA when consumption of highly palatable foods stops; thus, leading to increased motivation to continue addictive eating habits in an effort to mitigate the negative symptoms (Avena, Bocarsly, Hoebel, & Gold, 2011; Avena, Bocarsly, Rada, Kim, & Hoebel, 2008). This process is consistent with other substance addictions that maintain the addictive cycle through engagement in the addictive behavior, leading to satiation and tolerance, withdrawals and cravings, and continued use of the substance (Sussman & Sussman, 2011).

2.4 Food Cues

Mood states may differentially impact attention given to food cues in those with and without FA (Frayn, Sears, & von Ranson, 2016). Frayn et al. (2016) found that after inducing a sad mood, those with diagnosed FA (via YFAS) showed increased attention to unhealthy food cues compared to healthy controls. Functional neuroimaging studies consistently report that substance-related cues increase activation of reward networks involving the dorsolateral prefrontal cortex, orbitofrontal cortex, anterior cingulate cortex, amygdala, insula, and striatum and in addicted vs healthy subjects, assumed to contribute to continued use and relapse (Franklin et al., 2007; McBride, Barrett, Kelly, Aw, & Dagher, 2006). Conversely, when the desired substance is used, it typically leads to decreased reward circuit activation (Martinez et al., 2005, 2007; Volkow et al., 1997). This suggests that addicted individuals relative to healthy controls place a higher reward value on substance-related cues, but experience a lower level of satiation when the substance is used.

There is some indication that similar patterns exist in obese individuals when responding to food cues: these individuals show greater activation in the left dorsomedial prefrontal cortex, orbitofrontal cortex, right precentral gyrus, anterior cingulate cortex, amygdala, striatum, mediodorsal thalamus, and right parahippocampal gyrus (Brooks, Cedernaes, & Schioth, 2013; McBride et al., 2006). Like other drug-addicted individuals, those who are obese show less dorsal striatal and medial orbitofrontal cortex activation during the consumption of their "drug of choice" (Stice, Spoor, Bohon, & Small, 2008; Stice, Spoor, Bohon, Veldhuizen, & Small, 2008). As obesity is commonly associated with FA, it was hypothesized that similar activation patterns would be found in individuals who were diagnosed with a FA. Gearhardt, Yokum, et al. (2011) found that individuals who scored high on the YFAS (endorsed four or more items) showed activation in the left anterior cingulate cortex, left medial orbitofrontal cortex, and left amygdala when presented with a highly palatable food cue (ie, a chocolate milkshake solution administered through a syringe into the mouth of the subject while in the scanner), while those with low YFAS scores did not. Furthermore, the FA group showed decreased activation in the lateral orbitofrontal cortex during consumption of highly palatable food (Gearhardt, Yokum, et al., 2011). These results mirror those reported in research on other substance addictions, as well as those seen among obese individuals (Brooks et al., 2013). This provides evidence for a neurobiological mechanism underlying reward circuitry activation in individuals with FA.

2.5 Craving

Individuals with a high affinity for palatable foods have an increase in the strength of cravings when exposed to food cues (Stojek, Fischer, & MacKillop, 2015). Food craving for sweet or carbohydrate-rich foods was found to be a partial mediator between addictive eating and both elevated BMI and binge-eating episodes (Joyner, Gearhardt, & White, 2015), while cravings for high-fat foods appeared to mediate the relationship between addictive eating and elevated BMI (Joyner et al., 2015). Craving is a dynamic process, engaging reward, emotional, salience, self-referential, executive control, and memory networks (Ekhtiari, Nasseri, Yavari, Mokri, & Monterosso, 2016). A resting-state fMRI study showed increased functional connectivity between striatal reward network regions and self-referential default mode network regions (medial prefrontal cortex, posterior cingulate cortex, and angular gyrus), insula, and somatosensory cortex in overweight subjects (BMI > 25) relative to healthy controls. In addition, food-craving scores were positively correlated with the increased functional connectivity in the dorsal striatum (Contreras-Rodriguez, Martin-Perez, Vilar-Lopez, & Verdejo-Garcia, 2015). As suggested by the authors, the presence of increased connectivity in the dorsal striatal network observed in obese, but not normal weight subjects, provide evidence for neural adaptations in brain reward circuitry that may contribute to addictive eating. In addition to the striatum, brain reward regions usually associated with food cravings include the ventral tegmental area, nucleus accumbens, amygdala, and hippocampus (Frankort et al., 2014). Subjects given a monotonous diet for 1.5 days, consisting only of the complete nutrition drink "Boost," had greater brain activation in the insula, caudate, and hippocampus in response to cues of their favorite foods vs the monotonous food, ie, "Boost" (Pelchat, Johnson, Chan, Valdez, and Ragland (2004). The brain regions observed during cravings for favored foods overlapped with those seen for drug cravings, indicating that activation patterns of reward circuitry related to cravings may be similar in both FA and drug addiction (Volkow, Fowler, Wang, & Goldstein, 2002).

2.6 Impulsivity

Impulsivity, defined as an unplanned response to internal or external stimuli, without prior forethought and a disregard for potential negative consequences (Bari & Robbins, 2013), may account for reward-seeking behavior, and is associated with higher rates of relapse among addicted individuals (Doran, Spring, McChargue, Pergadia, & Richmond, 2004; Miller, 1991). Impulsivity includes difficulties with response inhibition and the inability to delay gratification, as evidenced by choosing an immediate reward over a long-term benefit (Winstanley, Eagle, & Robbins, 2006). Higher levels of impulsivity may be associated with hedonic eating (ie, eating after energy requirements have been met) patterns (Nederkoorn, Smulders, Havermans, Roefs, & Jansen, 2006). Impairments in impulse control mechanisms contribute to many disorders, including binge eating, bulimia nervosa, drug addiction, alcoholism, and Internet gaming (Alhassoon, Sorg, Stern,

Hall, & Wollman, 2015; Chen et al., 2016; Ding et al., 2014; Gearhardt, Boswell, & Potenza, 2014; Goldstein & Volkow, 2011).

Studies indicate that aberrant activities in regions such as the prefrontal cortex, anterior cingulate cortex, inferior frontal gyrus, and orbitofrontal cortex may be accompanied with impulsive behaviors (Davids et al., 2010; Tang, Posner, Rothbart, & Volkow, 2015; Uher et al., 2004). In a delay discounting task study, decreased activation of executive brain regions (ie, frontal gyri and inferior parietal lobule) in obese subjects was correlated to increased impulsivity as well as future weight gain (Kishinevsky et al., 2012; Stoeckel, Murdaugh, Cox, Cook, & Weller, 2013). These results suggest deficits of inhibitory functions in obese subjects. In addition, other self-regulatory control studies showed that people with bulimia nervosa had increased impulsivity with abnormal anterior cingulate and frontal cortical engagement (Marsh et al., 2011, 2009). Additional results suggest that those with disordered eating may have dysfunctional frontostriatal systems leading to a loss of control over feeding behavior. Deficient executive control, associated with impulsivity, as well as dysregulated craving and reward circuitry, may contribute to FA.

3. MAINTENANCE OF FA

3.1 Food Reward and Motivation

The mechanisms that contribute to maintaining FA are hypothesized to be similar to those in alcohol and illicit substance addictions (Avena et al., 2011; DiLeone, Taylor, & Picciotto, 2012; Hone-Blanchet & Fecteau, 2014). Similarities are primarily related to the effects these addictions have on the brain reward circuit (Parylak et al., 2011; Val-Laillet et al., 2015; Ziauddeen et al., 2015). The dopaminergic mesolimbic reward pathway connects the ventral tegmental area to the nucleus accumbens and is associated with positive reinforcement, food reward, and addiction (Volkow, Wang, Fowler, Tomasi, & Baler, 2012). Animal studies have shown that food has rewarding properties and can increase the firing rate of dopamine neurons and the release of dopamine in the nucleus accumbens (Hernandez & Hoebel, 1988; Norgren, Hajnal, & Mungarndee, 2006). Consumption of foods high in sugar content triggers the release of endogenous opioids in the nucleus accumbens, thus activating the dopaminergic reward system (Lerma-Cabrera, Carvajal, & Lopez-Legarrea, 2016). This mirrors the effects of other highly addictive substances, such as cocaine

(Blum, Thanos, & Gold, 2014) and speaks to the addictive potential of specific types of foods.

Substance addictions also show evidence of reward deficiency syndrome (Blum et al., 2000), a neural adaptation in response to continued exposure to a substance (or behavior, eg, gambling), that occurs when repeated engagement stimulates reward mechanisms so powerfully that the population of dopamine D2 receptors (D2R) declines (Benton & Young, 2016; Blum et al., 2000, 2014; Gyollai et al., 2014). Due to this decrease in D2R, increased intake is necessary in order to elicit the same degree of reward that was previously achieved through a lower dose (Blum et al., 2000). A further indication of the reward deficiency syndrome is the presence of intense cravings and withdrawal symptoms (Benton & Young, 2016). Similar reductions in D2Rs are hypothesized to occur in FA.

Benton and Young (2016) performed a meta-analysis to determine the relationship between BMI and the presence of Taq1A polymorphism, an A1 allele found to be associated with a lower number of D2R in both healthy and alcoholic subjects (Jonsson et al., 1999; Noble, Blum, Ritchie, Montgomery, & Sheridan, 1991; Pohjalainen et al., 1998). They found no significant effects of the A1 allele on BMI, and therefore concluded that there was no support for the reward deficiency theory of FA (Benton & Young, 2016). However, another study reported a negative correlation between BMI and the dorsal striatal response (left caudate, bilateral putamen) to a taste of chocolate milkshake vs water (Stice, Spoor, Bohon, et al., 2008): the presence of the A1 allele significantly moderated the negative correlation between BMI and left caudate activation. While additional studies are necessary to evaluate the reward deficiency hypothesis in FA, these results do demonstrate differing response levels in brain reward circuits related to consumption of highly palatable food in those with low vs high BMI's (Stice, Spoor, Bohon, et al., 2008). Specifically, the experience of reward from consuming food may not be as strong for those with higher BMI's, which may lead to overeating in an attempt to compensate for a dampened reward system.

3.2 Energy Homeostasis and Regulatory Mechanisms

Food intake is necessary for normal bodily energy expenditure, and appetite is controlled by complex neuronal and hormonal systems including the hypothalamus and peripheral satiety networks (Behary & Miras, 2014; Camilleri, 2015; Joly-Amado et al., 2014). Through a process known as "adiposity negative feedback," circulating signals from the body inform the brain of current energy stores. In response, the brain adjusts food intake (Kennedy, 1953). The hypothalamus is located directly below the thalamus in the limbic system and is responsible for a wide variety of regulatory functions, including body temperature, hunger, thirst, and the sleep–wake cycle (Snell, 2010). The peripheral satiety system includes hormonal inputs from the pancreas, liver, and adipose tissue (Morton, Meek, & Schwartz, 2014). Leptin is an adipocyte hormone that decreases appetite (as part of a negative feedback system) by acting on hypothalamic neurons that regulate energy homeostasis (Benoit, Clegg, Seeley, & Woods, 2004). Insulin, a pancreatic hormone much like leptin that it is sensitive to the amount of stored body fat, the levels of which increase when body fat is high and decrease when body fat is low, can also reduce appetite (Figlewicz, 2003). Ghrelin is a gustatory hormone that works to increase appetite (Chaudhri, Small, & Bloom, 2006; Kawahara et al., 2013; Wren & Bloom, 2007). It is believed that adiposity negative feedback works by increasing the brain's sensitivity to satiety signals (Morton et al., 2014). For example, as weight loss lowers plasma levels of leptin and insulin, the satiating effect of food is decreased. Conversely, as weight increases, these hormone levels also increase, producing a higher sensitivity to satiety signals (Hulsey, Lu, Wang, Martin, & Baile, 1998; Kahler et al., 1998). Communication between the hypothalamus and brain reward circuitry regulate these appetitive responses. For example, the lateral hypothalamic area receives information from the nucleus accumbens, allowing for the integration of information from reward brain regions and satiety signals from other areas of the central and peripheral nervous systems (Morton et al., 2005). This information is then projected to areas such as the hindbrain and the nucleus of the solitary tract, which are responsible for regulating satiety (Grill et al., 2002).

While leptin, insulin, and ghrelin work within the adiposity negative feedback system, other gut peptides are also involved in the perception of satiety and act as signals to increase or decrease appetite (Morton et al., 2014). Peptides that are implicated in reducing appetite include peptide YY (Batterham & Bloom, 2003), glucagon-like peptide 1 (van Bloemendaal, Ten Kulve, la Fleur, Ijzerman, & Diamant, 2014), and cholecystokinin (D'Agostino et al., 2016), and are secreted in response to food ingestion (Wren & Bloom, 2007). Mechanoreceptors located in the smooth muscle layer of the gut are also involved in sending satiety signals to the central nervous system, via afferent fibers along the vagus nerve that project to the nucleus of the solitary tract in the caudal hindbrain (Chaudhri et al., 2006; Morton et al., 2014). Other important components of appetite regulation include agouti-related protein receptors, located in the hypothalamic arcuate nucleus, which release neuropeptide Y, agouti-related peptide, and the neurotransmitter γ-aminobutyric acid (Krashes, Shah, Koda, & Lowell, 2013). Together, these work to promote appetite, when activated by ghrelin (Shrestha, Wickwire, & Giraudo, 2006), and are inhibited by insulin and leptin (Varela & Horvath, 2012).

Hypothalamic centers and peripheral networks strive to maintain homeostatic eating, defined as a state of equilibrium between the amount of energy taken in through food consumption and the metabolic demands of the body (Farr, Li, & Mantzoros, 2016). Over time, highly palatable foods may disrupt these appetite regulatory mechanisms (de Macedo et al., 2016; Johnson & Wardle, 2014) and promote hedonic eating (Lerma-Cabrera et al., 2016; Pandit, Mercer, Overduin, la Fleur, & Adan, 2012). Specifically, there is evidence that highly palatable foods can dampen satiety signals, thus leading to overeating. This is further compounded by increased activation of the reward system, which turns eating into a reward-driven behavior instead of a homeostatic process (Erlanson-Albertsson, 2005) (Fig. 1).

Prader Willi syndrome (PWS), a genetic disease that causes hypothalamic dysfunction, results in hyperphagia, obesity, stunted growth, and sleep abnormalities (Di Lorenzo, Sberveglieri, Marrama, Landi, & Ferri, 2016). Of particular interest to FA is the fact that those with PWS suffer from an insatiable appetite that often leads to overeating (McAllister, Whittington, & Holland, 2011). In individuals with PWS, the consumption of high calorie food is associated with significantly elevated activation of the orbitofrontal cortex and hypothalamus (Dimitropoulos & Schultz, 2008; Key & Dykens, 2008). In contrast to what is observed in healthy individuals—a decrease in ghrelin after a meal, terminating the motivation to consume more food (Chaudhri et al., 2006; Wren & Bloom, 2007)—those with PWS have increased ghrelin levels both before and after meals leading to overeating past the point of homeostatic energy demands (Feigerlova et al., 2008). Individuals with PWS are also likely to suffer from comorbid conditions, including anxiety and mood disorders (Hiraiwa, Maegaki, Oka, & Ohno, 2007), which as previously discussed are also associated with addictive eating (Singh, 2014).

3.3 The Impact of Stress on Hypothalamic Functioning

Chronic stress can independently contribute to addictive eating behaviors (Torres & Nowson, 2007). Recent models explaining the neuroadaptive

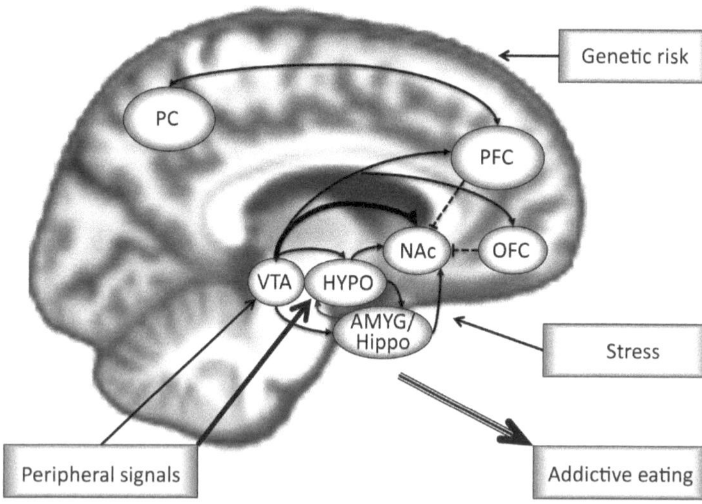

Fig. 1 Model of food addiction as a result of highly palpable food intake, stress, genetic risk, and overlapping circuits of the brain interacting with peripheral signals. The hypothalamus (HYPO) is part of the hypothalamic–pituitary–adrenal (HPA) axis, sensitive to stress, and critical for food intake. It is modulated by the ventral tegmental area (VTA) and amygdala (AMYG). In food addiction the strength of inhibitory control provided via orbitofrontal (OFC), prefrontal (PFC), and parietal cortices (PC) (*dashed lines*) is weakened and together with heightened food craving and seeking via reward VTA and nucleus accumbens (NAc) and addiction memory via limbic regions (AMYG/Hippocampus), and malfunctioning peripheral signals for appetite regulation (satiety), becomes a continued cycle of food addiction. *Adapted from DiLeone, R. J., Taylor, J. R., & Picciotto, M. R. (2012). The drive to eat: Comparisons and distinctions between mechanisms of food reward and drug addiction. Nature Neuroscience, 15 (10), 1330–1335. http://dx.doi.org/10.1038/nn.3202.*

consequences of acute and chronic stress responses now help explain the association between stress, addiction, and abnormal eating behaviors (Sinha & Jastreboff, 2013). Two systems, including the hypothalamic–pituitary–adrenal axis (HPA) and the autonomic nervous system, are responsible for physiological responses to acute stress (McEwen, 2007; Sinha, 2008). The HPA axis response commences with the release of corticotropin-releasing factor (CRF) from the paraventricular nucleus of the hypothalamus, which then triggers a release of adrenocorticotropin hormone (ACTH) from the anterior pituitary, resulting in the peripheral secretion of glucocorticoids, also known as cortisol or corticosterone, from the adrenal glands (McEwen, 2007). The release of CRF and ACTH helps with gluconeogenesis (Sinha & Jastreboff, 2013), which is a metabolic pathway responsible for generating glucose from noncarbohydrate substrates (Berg,

Tymoczko, & Stryer, 2002). These hormones also help with energy mobilization (Dallman, Akana, Strack, Hanson, & Sebastian, 1995), which is the process of directing and prioritizing stored energy, in the form of glucose, to parts of the body where it is most needed (Duffy, 1951). The release of CRF and ACTH during acute stress is terminated by glucocorticoid negative feedback, thereby allowing the systems to return to homeostasis (Dallman et al., 1995; Sinha & Jastreboff, 2013). Evidence from animal models indicates that during acute stress, food consumption decreases (Marti, Marti, & Armario, 1994), a result that has been replicated in human studies (Dallman, Pecoraro, & la Fleur, 2005).

After periods of prolonged and uncontrollable stress, the HPA axis can become dysregulated, leading to changes in the release patterns of hormones, neuropeptides, and glucocorticoids (Lupien, McEwen, Gunnar, & Heim, 2009; McEwen, 2007). Specifically, HPA axis dysregulation can cause insulin resistance due to altered glucose metabolism and can lead to excess abdominal fat (Wilcox, 2005). As levels of plasma insulin and abdominal fat increase, HPA axis activity decreases, and an increased intake of highly palatable foods is observed (Chrousos, 2000; Dallman et al., 2005; Tataranni et al., 1996; Warne, 2009). Stress-induced hypothalamic dysregulation may help explain the maintenance of FA (Berenson et al., 2015; Frayn et al., 2016; Micanti et al., 2016) (Fig. 1).

3.4 Cognitive Control and Addictive Eating

Cognitive control regions interact with reward and emotional systems, and act as top-down regulators to reorient attentional resources, make decisions, appraise rewards, and initiate or inhibit motivation to consume food (Ekhtiari, Faghiri, Oghabian, & Paulus, 2016; Schulte, Grilo, & Gearhardt, 2016; Spechler et al., 2016; Val-Laillet et al., 2015; Zilverstand, Parvaz, Moeller, & Goldstein, 2016). In obese populations, the consumption of highly palatable foods can lead to downregulation of the reward network, and deficiencies in cortical top-down regulation of eating behavior (Volkow, Wang, & Baler, 2011). In FA, the strength of inhibitory control provided via orbitofrontal, prefrontal, and parietal cortices is weakened and together with heightened food craving and seeking via the ventral tegmental area and nucleus accumbens, addiction memory via limbic regions (amygdala and hippocampus), and malfunctioning peripheral signals for appetite regulation (satiety), this becomes a vicious cycle (DiLeone et al., 2012) (see Fig. 1 for model).

4. DISCUSSION

The concept of "food addiction" is relatively novel, requires a clear definition, additional research, and a general consensus (Albayrak, Wolfle, & Hebebrand, 2012; Hebebrand et al., 2014; Ziauddeen et al., 2012; Ziauddeen & Fletcher, 2013). Proponents of the concept suggest that similarities between FA and other substance addictions, in particular, operant conditioning, effects of mood and stress, cue reactivity, craving, and impulsivity support food as an addictive substance (Ahmed et al., 2014; Berenson et al., 2015; Frayn et al., 2016; Kishinevsky et al., 2012; Pelchat et al., 2004). There is also some neural evidence supporting food as an addiction because of observations of downregulation of reward circuitry and difficulties with top-down cognitive control (Blum et al., 2014; Stice, Spoor, Bohon, et al., 2008; Volkow et al., 2003, 1997). Furthermore, animal studies show evidence of withdrawal symptoms in rats when access to sucrose solutions is terminated, as well as binge-like eating and dopaminergic dysregulation after removal of a high-fat diet (Avena et al., 2008; Carlin et al., 2016; Colantuoni et al., 2002). Critics of the FA hypothesis discuss an inability to pinpoint the exact "substance" that is responsible for the neuroaddictive responses (Ziauddeen & Fletcher, 2013). The types of foods involved in addictive eating are varied and even within one type of food, ie, carbohydrates, there are multiple chemicals and components (Ziauddeen et al., 2012; Ziauddeen & Fletcher, 2013). Moreover, those who deny the existence of FA claim there is not currently enough evidence that FA resembles other substance addictions from a neurological standpoint (Benton & Young, 2016; Ziauddeen & Fletcher, 2013).

However, there is evidence to support the notion that FA is an addiction according to the criteria put forth by Sussman and Sussman (2011). FA includes eating due to appetitive effects, preoccupation with food, temporary satiation, loss of control, and suffering negative consequences due to eating behaviors (Gearhardt, Boswell, & White, 2014; Gearhardt et al., 2016; Gearhardt, Yokum, et al., 2011; Joyner et al., 2015; Schulte, Grilo, & Gearhardt, 2016). FA does not, however, map perfectly onto a substance addiction model as purported in the DSM-5. Part of the problem is one of nomenclature: Hebebrand et al. (2014) suggest that "eating addiction" may better describe problematic hedonic eating than "food addiction," and in this sense, an eating addiction may be more similar to gambling disorder (American Psychiatric Association, 2013b). Gambling disorders have been found to affect brain reward circuitry in a manner similar to substance addiction, much like what is seen with FA. However, there is no "substance" causing the addiction (Blum et al., 2000; Gyollai et al., 2014).

While there may be considerable overlap with other abnormal eating patterns, there is a need to properly define FA criteria so as to better create representative experimental groups that will provide information on this condition in particular. The YFAS 2.0 has attempted to provide a framework for the diagnosis and grouping of individuals with FA. However, if FA were considered a behavioral addiction instead of a substance addiction, then the assessment would benefit from following a model more closely related to behavioral addictions in the DSM-5, such as gambling disorder, rather than the current model, which maps onto substance disorder criteria (American Psychiatric Association, 2013b; Hebebrand et al., 2014). Furthermore, the high prevalence of comorbid mental health disorders among addicted individuals, particularly involving mood dysregulation, may provide false positives on the YFAS 2.0 because many people eat in stressful situations or use eating to cope with negative affect (Albayrak et al., 2012). Efforts to disentangle FA from other eating disorders or health consequences related to eating, such as obesity and its associated negative influences on health, would help lend more credence to the concept of FA as a discrete condition.

ACKNOWLEDGMENTS

We thank Eden Gallanter and Eva M. Müller-Oehring for their critical review and comments on this manuscript. NIH Grant R01 AA023165 funded this work. The authors declare no conflict of interest.

REFERENCES

Ahmed, S., Kashem, M. A., Sarker, R., Ahmed, E. U., Hargreaves, G. A., & McGregor, I. S. (2014). Neuroadaptations in the striatal proteome of the rat following prolonged excessive sucrose intake. *Neurochemical Research*, *39*(5), 815–824. http://dx.doi.org/10.1007/s11064-014-1274-6.

Albayrak, O., Wolfle, S. M., & Hebebrand, J. (2012). Does food addiction exist? A phenomenological discussion based on the psychiatric classification of substance-related disorders and addiction. *Obesity Facts*, *5*(2), 165–179. http://dx.doi.org/10.1159/000338310.

Alhassoon, O. M., Sorg, S. F., Stern, M. J., Hall, M. G., & Wollman, S. C. (2015). Neuroimaging in alcohol-use disorders: Clinical implications and future directions. *Future Neurology*, *10*(4), 345–356. http://dx.doi.org/10.2217/fnl.15.17.

American Psychiatric Association (2013a). *Feeding and eating disorders diagnostic and statistical manual of mental disorders* (5th ed.). Washington, DC: American Psychiatric Association.

American Psychiatric Association (2013b). *Substance-related and addictive disorders diagnostic and statistical manual of mental disorders* (5th ed.). Washington, DC: American Psychiatric Association.

Avena, N. M., Bocarsly, M. E., Hoebel, B. G., & Gold, M. S. (2011). Overlaps in the nosology of substance abuse and overeating: The translational implications of "food addiction". *Current Drug Abuse Reviews*, *4*(3), 133–139.

Avena, N. M., Bocarsly, M. E., Rada, P., Kim, A., & Hoebel, B. G. (2008). After daily bingeing on a sucrose solution, food deprivation induces anxiety and accumbens dopamine/acetylcholine imbalance. *Physiology & Behavior*, *94*(3), 309–315. http://dx.doi.org/10.1016/j.physbeh.2008.01.008.

Bari, A., & Robbins, T. W. (2013). Inhibition and impulsivity: Behavioral and neural basis of response control. *Progress in Neurobiology*, *108*, 44–79. http://dx.doi.org/10.1016/j.pneurobio.2013.06.005.

Batterham, R. L., & Bloom, S. R. (2003). The gut hormone peptide YY regulates appetite. *Annals of the New York Academy of Sciences*, *994*, 162–168.

Behary, P., & Miras, A. D. (2014). Brain responses to food and weight loss. *Experimental Physiology*, *99*(9), 1121–1127. http://dx.doi.org/10.1113/expphysiol.2014.078303.

Benoit, S. C., Clegg, D. J., Seeley, R. J., & Woods, S. C. (2004). Insulin and leptin as adiposity signals. *Recent Progress in Hormone Research*, *59*, 267–285.

Benton, D., & Young, H. A. (2016). A meta-analysis of the relationship between brain dopamine receptors and obesity: A matter of changes in behavior rather than food addiction? *International Journal of Obesity (London)*, *40*(Suppl. 1), S12–S21. http://dx.doi.org/10.1038/ijo.2016.9.

Berenson, A. B., Laz, T. H., Pohlmeier, A. M., Rahman, M., & Cunningham, K. A. (2015). Prevalence of food addiction among low-income reproductive-aged women. *Journal of Women's Health (2002)*, *24*(9), 740–744. http://dx.doi.org/10.1089/jwh.2014.5182.

Berg, J. M., Tymoczko, J. L., & Stryer, L. (2002). *Biochemistry, glycolysis and gluconeogenesis.* New York: WH Freeman. Retrieved from. http://www.ncbi.nlm.nih.gov/books/NBK21150/.

Blum, K., Braverman, E. R., Holder, J. M., Lubar, J. F., Monastra, V. J., Miller, D., … Comings, D. E. (2000). Reward deficiency syndrome: A biogenetic model for the diagnosis and treatment of impulsive, addictive, and compulsive behaviors. *Journal of Psychoactive Drugs*, *32*(Suppl. i–iv), 1–112.

Blum, K., Thanos, P. K., & Gold, M. S. (2014). Dopamine and glucose, obesity, and reward deficiency syndrome. *Frontiers in Psychology*, *5*, 919. http://dx.doi.org/10.3389/fpsyg.2014.00919.

Brooks, S. J., Cedernaes, J., & Schioth, H. B. (2013). Increased prefrontal and parahippocampal activation with reduced dorsolateral prefrontal and insular cortex activation to food images in obesity: A meta-analysis of fMRI studies. *PloS One*, *8*(4), e60393. http://dx.doi.org/10.1371/journal.pone.0060393.

Camilleri, M. (2015). Peripheral mechanisms in appetite regulation. *Gastroenterology*, *148*(6), 1219–1233. http://dx.doi.org/10.1053/j.gastro.2014.09.016.

Carlin, J. L., McKee, S. E., Hill-Smith, T., Grissom, N. M., George, R., Lucki, I., & Reyes, T. M. (2016). Removal of high-fat diet after chronic exposure drives binge behavior and dopaminergic dysregulation in female mice. *Neuroscience*, *326*, 170–179. http://dx.doi.org/10.1016/j.neuroscience.2016.04.002.

Chaudhri, O., Small, C., & Bloom, S. (2006). Gastrointestinal hormones regulating appetite. *Philosophical Transactions of the Royal Society of London. Series B, Biological Sciences*, *361*(1471), 1187–1209. http://dx.doi.org/10.1098/rstb.2006.1856.

Chen, C. Y., Yen, J. Y., Wang, P. W., Liu, G. C., Yen, C. F., & Ko, C. H. (2016). Altered functional connectivity of the insula and nucleus accumbens in internet gaming disorder: A resting state fMRI study. *European Addiction Research*, *22*(4), 192–200. http://dx.doi.org/10.1159/000440716.

Chrousos, G. P. (2000). The stress response and immune function: Clinical implications. The 1999 Novera H. Spector lecture. *Annals of the New York Academy of Sciences*, *917*, 38–67.

Colantuoni, C., Rada, P., McCarthy, J., Patten, C., Avena, N. M., Chadeayne, A., & Hoebel, B. G. (2002). Evidence that intermittent, excessive sugar intake causes endogenous opioid dependence. *Obesity Research*, *10*(6), 478–488. http://dx.doi.org/10.1038/oby.2002.66.

Contreras-Rodriguez, O., Martin-Perez, C., Vilar-Lopez, R., & Verdejo-Garcia, A. (2015). Ventral and dorsal striatum networks in obesity: Link to food craving and weight gain. *Biological Psychiatry*. http://dx.doi.org/10.1016/j.biopsych.2015.11.020. (Epub ahead of print).

Cui, C., Noronha, A., Morikawa, H., Alvarez, V. A., Stuber, G. D., Szumlinski, K. K., … Wilcox, M. V. (2013). New insights on neurobiological mechanisms underlying alcohol addiction. *Neuropharmacology*, *67*, 223–232. http://dx.doi.org/10.1016/j.neuropharm.2012.09.022.

D'Agostino, G., Lyons, D. J., Cristiano, C., Burke, L. K., Madara, J. C., Campbell, J. N., … Heisler, L. K. (2016). Appetite controlled by a cholecystokinin nucleus of the solitary tract to hypothalamus neurocircuit. *Elife*, *5*, e12225, http://dx.doi.org/10.7554/eLife.12225.

Dallman, M. F., Akana, S. F., Strack, A. M., Hanson, E. S., & Sebastian, R. J. (1995). The neural network that regulates energy balance is responsive to glucocorticoids and insulin and also regulates HPA axis responsivity at a site proximal to CRF neurons. *Annals of the New York Academy of Sciences*, *771*, 730–742.

Dallman, M. F., Pecoraro, N. C., & la Fleur, S. E. (2005). Chronic stress and comfort foods: Self-medication and abdominal obesity. *Brain, Behavior, and Immunity*, *19*(4), 275–280. http://dx.doi.org/10.1016/j.bbi.2004.11.004.

Davids, S., Lauffer, H., Thoms, K., Jagdhuhn, M., Hirschfeld, H., Domin, M., … Lotze, M. (2010). Increased dorsolateral prefrontal cortex activation in obese children during observation of food stimuli. *International Journal of Obesity*, *34*(1), 94–104. http://dx.doi.org/10.1038/ijo.2009.193.

Davis, C., Curtis, C., Levitan, R. D., Carter, J. C., Kaplan, A. S., & Kennedy, J. L. (2011). Evidence that 'food addiction' is a valid phenotype of obesity. *Appetite*, *57*(3), 711–717. http://dx.doi.org/10.1016/j.appet.2011.08.017.

de Macedo, I. C., de Freitas, J. S., & da Silva Torres, I. L. (2016). The influence of palatable diets in reward system activation: A mini review. *Advances in Pharmacological Sciences*, *2016*, 7238679. http://dx.doi.org/10.1155/2016/7238679.

Di Lorenzo, R., Sberveglieri, S., Marrama, D., Landi, G., & Ferri, P. (2016). Weight control and behavior rehabilitation in a patient suffering from Prader Willi syndrome. *BMC Research Notes*, *9*(1), 199. http://dx.doi.org/10.1186/s13104-016-1981-y.

DiLeone, R. J., Taylor, J. R., & Picciotto, M. R. (2012). The drive to eat: Comparisons and distinctions between mechanisms of food reward and drug addiction. *Nature Neuroscience*, *15*(10), 1330–1335. http://dx.doi.org/10.1038/nn.3202.

Dimitropoulos, A., & Schultz, R. T. (2008). Food-related neural circuitry in Prader-Willi syndrome: Response to high- versus low-calorie foods. *Journal of Autism and Developmental Disorders*, *38*(9), 1642–1653. http://dx.doi.org/10.1007/s10803-008-0546-x.

Ding, W. N., Sun, J. H., Sun, Y. W., Chen, X., Zhou, Y., Zhuang, Z. G., … Du, Y. S. (2014). Trait impulsivity and impaired prefrontal impulse inhibition function in adolescents with internet gaming addiction revealed by a Go/No-Go fMRI study. *Behavioral and Brain Functions*, *10*, 20. http://dx.doi.org/10.1186/1744-9081-10-20.

Doran, N., Spring, B., McChargue, D., Pergadia, M., & Richmond, M. (2004). Impulsivity and smoking relapse. *Nicotine & Tobacco Research*, *6*(4), 641–647. http://dx.doi.org/10.1080/14622200410001727939.

Duffy, E. (1951). The concept of energy mobilization. *Psychological Review*, *58*(1), 30–40.

Ekhtiari, H., Faghiri, A., Oghabian, M.-A., & Paulus, M. P. (2016). Functional neuroimaging for addiction medicine: From mechanisms to practical considerations. In E. Hamed & P. P. Martin (Eds.), *Progress in Brain Research. : Vol. 224.* (pp. 129–153). Cambridge, MA: Elsevier. chapter 7.

Ekhtiari, H., Nasseri, P., Yavari, F., Mokri, A., & Monterosso, J. (2016). Neuroscience of drug craving for addiction medicine: From circuits to therapies. In E. Hamed & P. Martin (Eds.), *Progress in brain research: Vol. 223.* (pp. 115–141). Cambridge, MA: Elsevier. chapter 7.

Erlanson-Albertsson, C. (2005). How palatable food disrupts appetite regulation. *Basic & Clinical Pharmacology & Toxicology, 97*(2), 61–73. http://dx.doi.org/10.1111/j.1742-7843.2005.pto_179.x.

Farr, O. M., Li, C. S., & Mantzoros, C. S. (2016). Central nervous system regulation of eating: Insights from human brain imaging. *Metabolism, 65*(5), 699–713. http://dx.doi.org/10.1016/j.metabol.2016.02.002.

Feigerlova, E., Diene, G., Conte-Auriol, F., Molinas, C., Gennero, I., Salles, J. P., … Tauber, M. (2008). Hyperghrelinemia precedes obesity in Prader-Willi syndrome. *The Journal of Clinical Endocrinology and Metabolism, 93*(7), 2800–2805. http://dx.doi.org/10.1210/jc.2007-2138.

Figlewicz, D. P. (2003). Adiposity signals and food reward: Expanding the CNS roles of insulin and leptin. *American Journal of Physiology. Regulatory, Integrative and Comparative Physiology, 284*(4), R882–R892. http://dx.doi.org/10.1152/ajpregu.00602.2002.

Franklin, T. R., Wang, Z., Wang, J., Sciortino, N., Harper, D., Li, Y., … Childress, A. R. (2007). Limbic activation to cigarette smoking cues independent of nicotine withdrawal: A perfusion fMRI study. *Neuropsychopharmacology, 32*(11), 2301–2309. http://dx.doi.org/10.1038/sj.npp.1301371.

Frankort, A., Roefs, A., Siep, N., Roebroeck, A., Havermans, R., & Jansen, A. (2014). The craving stops before you feel it: Neural correlates of chocolate craving during cue exposure with response prevention. *Cerebral Cortex, 24*(6), 1589–1600. http://dx.doi.org/10.1093/cercor/bht016.

Frayn, M., Sears, C. R., & von Ranson, K. M. (2016). A sad mood increases attention to unhealthy food images in women with food addiction. *Appetite, 100*, 55–63. http://dx.doi.org/10.1016/j.appet.2016.02.008.

Gearhardt, A. N., Boswell, R. G., & Potenza, M. N. (2014a). Neuroimaging of eating disorders, substance use disorders, and addictions: Overlapping and unique systems. In D. T. Brewerton & A. Baker Dennis (Eds.), *Eating disorders, addictions and substance use disorders: Research, clinical and treatment perspectives* (pp. 71–89). Berlin, Heidelberg: Springer.

Gearhardt, A. N., Boswell, R. G., & White, M. A. (2014b). The association of "food addiction" with disordered eating and body mass index. *Eating Behaviors, 15*(3), 427–433. http://dx.doi.org/10.1016/j.eatbeh.2014.05.001.

Gearhardt, A. N., Corbin, W. R., & Brownell, K. D. (2016). Development of the Yale Food Addiction Scale Version 2.0. *Psychology of Addictive Behaviors, 30*(1), 113–121. http://dx.doi.org/10.1037/adb0000136.

Gearhardt, A. N., Davis, C., Kuschner, R., & Brownell, K. D. (2011). The addiction potential of hyperpalatable foods. *Current Drug Abuse Reviews, 4*(3), 140–145.

Gearhardt, A. N., Grilo, C. M., DiLeone, R. J., Brownell, K. D., & Potenza, M. N. (2011). Can food be addictive? Public health and policy implications. *Addiction, 106*(7), 1208–1212. http://dx.doi.org/10.1111/j.1360-0443.2010.03301.x.

Gearhardt, A. N., Yokum, S., Orr, P. T., Stice, E., Corbin, W. R., & Brownell, K. D. (2011). Neural correlates of food addiction. *Archives of General Psychiatry, 68*(8), 808–816. http://dx.doi.org/10.1001/archgenpsychiatry.2011.32.

Geliebter, A., & Aversa, A. (2003). Emotional eating in overweight, normal weight, and underweight individuals. *Eating Behaviors, 3*(4), 341–347.

Giuliani, N. R., & Pfeifer, J. H. (2015). Age-related changes in reappraisal of appetitive cravings during adolescence. *NeuroImage*, *108*, 173–181. http://dx.doi.org/10.1016/j.neuroimage.2014.12.037.

Goldschmidt, A. B., Wall, M., Choo, T. H., Becker, C., & Neumark-Sztainer, D. (2016). Shared risk factors for mood-, eating-, and weight-related health outcomes. *Health Psychology*, *35*(3), 245–252. http://dx.doi.org/10.1037/hea0000283.

Goldstein, R. Z., & Volkow, N. D. (2011). Dysfunction of the prefrontal cortex in addiction: Neuroimaging findings and clinical implications. *Nature Reviews. Neuroscience*, *12*(11), 652–669. http://dx.doi.org/10.1038/nrn3119.

Grill, H. J., Schwartz, M. W., Kaplan, J. M., Foxhall, J. S., Breininger, J., & Baskin, D. G. (2002). Evidence that the caudal brainstem is a target for the inhibitory effect of leptin on food intake. *Endocrinology*, *143*(1), 239–246. http://dx.doi.org/10.1210/endo.143.1.8589.

Gyollai, A., Griffiths, M. D., Barta, C., Vereczkei, A., Urban, R., Kun, B., … Demetrovics, Z. (2014). The genetics of problem and pathological gambling: A systematic review. *Current Pharmaceutical Design*, *20*(25), 3993–3999.

Hebebrand, J., Albayrak, O., Adan, R., Antel, J., Dieguez, C., de Jong, J., … Dickson, S. L. (2014). "Eating addiction", rather than "food addiction", better captures addictive-like eating behavior. *Neuroscience and Biobehavioral Reviews*, *47*, 295–306. http://dx.doi.org/10.1016/j.neubiorev.2014.08.016.

Hernandez, L., & Hoebel, B. G. (1988). Food reward and cocaine increase extracellular dopamine in the nucleus accumbens as measured by microdialysis. *Life Sciences*, *42*(18), 1705–1712.

Hiraiwa, R., Maegaki, Y., Oka, A., & Ohno, K. (2007). Behavioral and psychiatric disorders in Prader-Willi syndrome: A population study in Japan. *Brain and Development*, *29*(9), 535–542. http://dx.doi.org/10.1016/j.braindev.2007.01.005.

Hone-Blanchet, A., & Fecteau, S. (2014). Overlap of food addiction and substance use disorders definitions: Analysis of animal and human studies. *Neuropharmacology*, *85*, 81–90. http://dx.doi.org/10.1016/j.neuropharm.2014.05.019.

Huerta, C. I., Sarkar, P. R., Duong, T. Q., Laird, A. R., & Fox, P. T. (2014). Neural bases of food perception: Coordinate-based meta-analyses of neuroimaging studies in multiple modalities. *Obesity (Silver Spring)*, *22*(6), 1439–1446. http://dx.doi.org/10.1002/oby.20659.

Hulsey, M. G., Lu, H., Wang, T., Martin, R. J., & Baile, C. A. (1998). Intracerebroventricular (i.c.v.) administration of mouse leptin in rats: Behavioral specificity and effects on meal patterns. *Physiology & Behavior*, *65*(3), 445–455.

Jiang, T., Soussignan, R., Schaal, B., & Royet, J. P. (2015). Reward for food odors: An fMRI study of liking and wanting as a function of metabolic state and BMI. *Social Cognitive and Affective Neuroscience*, *10*(4), 561–568. http://dx.doi.org/10.1093/scan/nsu086.

Johnson, P. M., & Kenny, P. J. (2010). Dopamine D2 receptors in addiction-like reward dysfunction and compulsive eating in obese rats. *Nature Neuroscience*, *13*(5), 635–641. http://dx.doi.org/10.1038/nn.2519.

Johnson, F., & Wardle, J. (2014). Variety, palatability, and obesity. *Advances in Nutrition*, *5*(6), 851–859. http://dx.doi.org/10.3945/an.114.007120.

Joly-Amado, A., Cansell, C., Denis, R. G., Delbes, A. S., Castel, J., Martinez, S., & Luquet, S. (2014). The hypothalamic arcuate nucleus and the control of peripheral substrates. *Best Practice & Research. Clinical Endocrinology & Metabolism*, *28*(5), 725–737. http://dx.doi.org/10.1016/j.beem.2014.03.003.

Jonsson, E. G., Nothen, M. M., Grunhage, F., Farde, L., Nakashima, Y., Propping, P., & Sedvall, G. C. (1999). Polymorphisms in the dopamine D2 receptor gene and their relationships to striatal dopamine receptor density of healthy volunteers. *Molecular Psychiatry*, *4*(3), 290–296.

Joyner, M. A., Gearhardt, A. N., & White, M. A. (2015). Food craving as a mediator between addictive-like eating and problematic eating outcomes. *Eating Behaviors*, *19*, 98–101. http://dx.doi.org/10.1016/j.eatbeh.2015.07.005.

Kahler, A., Geary, N., Eckel, L. A., Campfield, L. A., Smith, F. J., & Langhans, W. (1998). Chronic administration of OB protein decreases food intake by selectively reducing meal size in male rats. *The American Journal of Physiology*, *275*(1 Pt. 2), R180–R185.

Kawahara, Y., Kaneko, F., Yamada, M., Kishikawa, Y., Kawahara, H., & Nishi, A. (2013). Food reward-sensitive interaction of ghrelin and opioid receptor pathways in mesolimbic dopamine system. *Neuropharmacology*, *67*, 395–402. http://dx.doi.org/10.1016/j.neuropharm.2012.11.022.

Kelly, A. C., Vimalakanthan, K., & Carter, J. C. (2014). Understanding the roles of self-esteem, self-compassion, and fear of self-compassion in eating disorder pathology: An examination of female students and eating disorder patients. *Eating Behaviors*, *15*(3), 388–391. http://dx.doi.org/10.1016/j.eatbeh.2014.04.008.

Kennedy, G. C. (1953). The role of depot fat in the hypothalamic control of food intake in the rat. *Proceedings of the Royal Society of London - Series B: Biological Sciences*, *140*(901), 578–596.

Key, A. P., & Dykens, E. M. (2008). 'Hungry eyes': Visual processing of food images in adults with Prader-Willi syndrome. *Journal of Intellectual Disability Research*, *52*(Pt. 6), 536–546. http://dx.doi.org/10.1111/j.1365-2788.2008.01062.x.

Kishinevsky, F. I., Cox, J. E., Murdaugh, D. L., Stoeckel, L. E., Cook, E. W., 3rd., & Weller, R. E. (2012). fMRI reactivity on a delay discounting task predicts weight gain in obese women. *Appetite*, *58*(2), 582–592. http://dx.doi.org/10.1016/j.appet. 2011.11.029.

Koob, G. F. (2000). Neurobiology of addiction. Toward the development of new therapies. *Annals of the New York Academy of Sciences*, *909*, 170–185.

Koob, G. F. (2003). Neuroadaptive mechanisms of addiction: Studies on the extended amygdala. *European Neuropsychopharmacology*, *13*(6), 442–452.

Koob, G. F. (2013). Theoretical frameworks and mechanistic aspects of alcohol addiction: Alcohol addiction as a reward deficit disorder. *Current Topics in Behavioral Neurosciences*, *13*, 3–30. http://dx.doi.org/10.1007/7854_2011_129.

Krashes, M. J., Shah, B. P., Koda, S., & Lowell, B. B. (2013). Rapid versus delayed stimulation of feeding by the endogenously released AgRP neuron mediators GABA, NPY, and AgRP. *Cell Metabolism*, *18*(4), 588–595. http://dx.doi.org/10.1016/j.cmet.2013. 09.009.

Lao-Kaim, N. P., Fonville, L., Giampietro, V. P., Williams, S. C., Simmons, A., & Tchanturia, K. (2015). Aberrant function of learning and cognitive control networks underlie inefficient cognitive flexibility in anorexia nervosa: A cross-sectional fMRI study. *PloS One*, *10*(5), e0124027. http://dx.doi.org/10.1371/journal.pone.0124027.

Lerma-Cabrera, J. M., Carvajal, F., & Lopez-Legarrea, P. (2016). Food addiction as a new piece of the obesity framework. *Nutrition Journal*, *15*, 5. http://dx.doi.org/10.1186/s12937-016-0124-6.

Lupien, S. J., McEwen, B. S., Gunnar, M. R., & Heim, C. (2009). Effects of stress throughout the lifespan on the brain, behaviour and cognition. *Nature Reviews. Neuroscience*, *10*(6), 434–445. http://dx.doi.org/10.1038/nrn2639.

Marsh, R., Horga, G., Wang, Z., Wang, P., Klahr, K. W., Berner, L. A., … Peterson, B. S. (2011). An FMRI study of self-regulatory control and conflict resolution in adolescents with bulimia nervosa. *The American Journal of Psychiatry*, *168*(11), 1210–1220. http://dx.doi.org/10.1176/appi.ajp.2011.11010094.

Marsh, R., Steinglass, J. E., Gerber, A. J., Graziano O'Leary, K., Wang, Z., Murphy, D., … Peterson, B. S. (2009). Deficient activity in the neural systems that mediate self-regulatory control in bulimia nervosa. *Archives of General Psychiatry*, *66*(1), 51–63. http://dx.doi.org/10.1001/archgenpsychiatry.2008.504.

Marti, O., Marti, J., & Armario, A. (1994). Effects of chronic stress on food intake in rats: Influence of stressor intensity and duration of daily exposure. *Physiology & Behavior, 55*(4), 747–753.

Martinez, D., Gil, R., Slifstein, M., Hwang, D. R., Huang, Y., Perez, A., … Abi-Dargham, A. (2005). Alcohol dependence is associated with blunted dopamine transmission in the ventral striatum. *Biological Psychiatry, 58*(10), 779–786. http://dx.doi.org/10.1016/j.biopsych.2005.04.044.

Martinez, D., Narendran, R., Foltin, R. W., Slifstein, M., Hwang, D. R., Broft, A., … Laruelle, M. (2007). Amphetamine-induced dopamine release: Markedly blunted in cocaine dependence and predictive of the choice to self-administer cocaine. *The American Journal of Psychiatry, 164*(4), 622–629. http://dx.doi.org/10.1176/ajp.2007.164.4.622.

McAllister, C. J., Whittington, J. E., & Holland, A. J. (2011). Development of the eating behaviour in Prader-Willi syndrome: Advances in our understanding. *International Journal of Obesity, 35*(2), 188–197. http://dx.doi.org/10.1038/ijo.2010.139.

McBride, D., Barrett, S. P., Kelly, J. T., Aw, A., & Dagher, A. (2006). Effects of expectancy and abstinence on the neural response to smoking cues in cigarette smokers: An fMRI study. *Neuropsychopharmacology, 31*(12), 2728–2738. http://dx.doi.org/10.1038/sj.npp.1301075.

McEwen, B. S. (2007). Physiology and neurobiology of stress and adaptation: Central role of the brain. *Physiological Reviews, 87*(3), 873–904. http://dx.doi.org/10.1152/physrev.00041.2006.

Meule, A. (2011). How prevalent is "food addiction"? *Frontiers in Psychology, 2*, 61. http://dx.doi.org/10.3389/fpsyt.2011.00061.

Meule, A. (2015). Back by popular demand: A narrative review on the history of food addiction research. *The Yale Journal of Biology and Medicine, 88*(3), 295–302.

Meule, A., & Kubler, A. (2012). Food cravings in food addiction: The distinct role of positive reinforcement. *Eating Behaviors, 13*(3), 252–255. http://dx.doi.org/10.1016/j.eatbeh.2012.02.001.

Micanti, F., Iasevoli, F., Cucciniello, C., Costabile, R., Loiarro, G., Pecoraro, G., … Galletta, D. (2016). The relationship between emotional regulation and eating behaviour: A multidimensional analysis of obesity psychopathology. *Eating and Weight Disorders*. http://dx.doi.org/10.1007/s40519-016-0275-7. (Epub ahead of print).

Miller, L. (1991). Predicting relapse and recovery in alcoholism and addiction: Neuropsychology, personality, and cognitive style. *Journal of Substance Abuse Treatment, 8*(4), 277–291.

Monro, J. A., & Shaw, M. (2008). Glycemic impact, glycemic glucose equivalents, glycemic index, and glycemic load: Definitions, distinctions, and implications. *The American Journal of Clinical Nutrition, 87*(1), 237S–243S.

Morton, G. J., Blevins, J. E., Williams, D. L., Niswender, K. D., Gelling, R. W., Rhodes, C. J., … Schwartz, M. W. (2005). Leptin action in the forebrain regulates the hindbrain response to satiety signals. *The Journal of Clinical Investigation, 115*(3), 703–710. http://dx.doi.org/10.1172/JCI22081.

Morton, G. J., Meek, T. H., & Schwartz, M. W. (2014). Neurobiology of food intake in health and disease. *Nature Reviews. Neuroscience, 15*(6), 367–378. http://dx.doi.org/10.1038/nrn3745.

Murdaugh, D. L., Cox, J. E., Cook, E. W., 3rd., & Weller, R. E. (2012). fMRI reactivity to high-calorie food pictures predicts short- and long-term outcome in a weight-loss program. *NeuroImage, 59*(3), 2709–2721.

National Institutes of Health & Department of Health and Human Services. Assessing your weight and health risk. Retrieved May 24, 2016, from http://www.nhlbi.nih.gov/health/educational/lose_wt/risk.htm.

Nederkoorn, C., Smulders, F. T., Havermans, R. C., Roefs, A., & Jansen, A. (2006). Impulsivity in obese women. *Appetite*, *47*(2), 253–256. http://dx.doi.org/10.1016/j.appet.2006.05.008.
Noble, E. P., Blum, K., Ritchie, T., Montgomery, A., & Sheridan, P. J. (1991). Allelic association of the D2 dopamine receptor gene with receptor-binding characteristics in alcoholism. *Archives of General Psychiatry*, *48*(7), 648–654.
Norgren, R., Hajnal, A., & Mungarndee, S. S. (2006). Gustatory reward and the nucleus accumbens. *Physiology & Behavior*, *89*(4), 531–535. http://dx.doi.org/10.1016/j.physbeh.2006.05.024.
Pandit, R., Mercer, J. G., Overduin, J., la Fleur, S. E., & Adan, R. A. (2012). Dietary factors affect food reward and motivation to eat. *Obesity Facts*, *5*(2), 221–242. http://dx.doi.org/10.1159/000338073.
Parylak, S. L., Koob, G. F., & Zorrilla, E. P. (2011). The dark side of food addiction. *Physiology & Behavior*, *104*(1), 149–156. http://dx.doi.org/10.1016/j.physbeh.2011.04.063.
Pelchat, M. L., Johnson, A., Chan, R., Valdez, J., & Ragland, J. D. (2004). Images of desire: Food-craving activation during fMRI. *NeuroImage*, *23*(4), 1486–1493. http://dx.doi.org/10.1016/j.neuroimage.2004.08.023.
Pohjalainen, T., Rinne, J. O., Nagren, K., Lehikoinen, P., Anttila, K., Syvalahti, E. K., & Hietala, J. (1998). The A1 allele of the human D2 dopamine receptor gene predicts low D2 receptor availability in healthy volunteers. *Molecular Psychiatry*, *3*(3), 256–260.
Pursey, K. M., Stanwell, P., Gearhardt, A. N., Collins, C. E., & Burrows, T. L. (2014). The prevalence of food addiction as assessed by the Yale Food Addiction Scale: A systematic review. *Nutrients*, *6*(10), 4552–4590. http://dx.doi.org/10.3390/nu6104552.
Robinson, M. J., Fischer, A. M., Ahuja, A., Lesser, E. N., & Maniates, H. (2016). Roles of "wanting" and "liking" in motivating behavior: Gambling, food, and drug addictions. *Current Topics in Behavioral Neurosciences*, *27*, 105–136. http://dx.doi.org/10.1007/7854_2015_387.
Rolls, E. T. (2015). Taste, olfactory, and food reward value processing in the brain. *Progress in Neurobiology*, *127–128*, 64–90. http://dx.doi.org/10.1016/j.pneurobio.2015.03.002.
Rolls, E. T., Kellerhals, M. B., & Nichols, T. E. (2015). Age differences in the brain mechanisms of good taste. *NeuroImage*, *113*, 298–309. http://dx.doi.org/10.1016/j.neuroimage.2015.03.065.
Schulte, E. M., Avena, N. M., & Gearhardt, A. N. (2015). Which foods may be addictive? The roles of processing, fat content, and glycemic load. *PloS One*, *10*(2), e0117959. http://dx.doi.org/10.1371/journal.pone.0117959.
Schulte, E. M., Grilo, C. M., & Gearhardt, A. N. (2016). Shared and unique mechanisms underlying binge eating disorder and addictive disorders. *Clinical Psychology Review*, *44*, 125–139. http://dx.doi.org/10.1016/j.cpr.2016.02.001.
Shrestha, Y. B., Wickwire, K., & Giraudo, S. Q. (2006). Role of AgRP on Ghrelin-induced feeding in the hypothalamic paraventricular nucleus. *Regulatory Peptides*, *133*(1–3), 68–73. http://dx.doi.org/10.1016/j.regpep.2005.09.021.
Simmons, W. K., Rapuano, K. M., Ingeholm, J. E., Avery, J., Kallman, S., Hall, K. D., & Martin, A. (2014). The ventral pallidum and orbitofrontal cortex support food pleasantness inferences. *Brain Structure & Function*, *219*(2), 473–483. http://dx.doi.org/10.1007/s00429-013-0511-0.
Simon, J. J., Skunde, M., Walther, S., Bendszus, M., Herzog, W., & Friederich, H. C. (2016). Neural signature of food reward processing in bulimic-type eating disorders. *Social Cognitive and Affective Neuroscience*. http://dx.doi.org/10.1093/scan/nsw049. (Epub ahead of print).
Singh, M. (2014). Mood, food, and obesity. *Frontiers in Psychology*, *5*, 925. http://dx.doi.org/10.3389/fpsyg.2014.00925.

Sinha, R. (2008). Chronic stress, drug use, and vulnerability to addiction. *Annals of the New York Academy of Sciences, 1141*, 105–130. http://dx.doi.org/10.1196/annals.1441.030.

Sinha, R., & Jastreboff, A. M. (2013). Stress as a common risk factor for obesity and addiction. *Biological Psychiatry, 73*(9), 827–835. http://dx.doi.org/10.1016/j.biopsych.2013.01.032.

Snell, R. S. (2010). *Clinical neuroanatomy*. Philadelphia: Lippincott Williams.

Spanagel, R., Noori, H. R., & Heilig, M. (2014). Stress and alcohol interactions: Animal studies and clinical significance. *Trends in Neurosciences, 37*(4), 219–227. http://dx.doi.org/10.1016/j.tins.2014.02.006.

Spechler, P. A., Chaarani, B., Hudson, K. E., Potter, A., Foxe, J. J., & Garavan, H. (2016). Response inhibition and addiction medicine: From use to abstinence. In E. Hamed & P. Martin (Eds.), *Progress in brain research: Vol. 223*. (pp. 143–164). Cambridge, MA: Elsevier. chapter 8.

Stice, E., Spoor, S., Bohon, C., & Small, D. M. (2008a). Relation between obesity and blunted striatal response to food is moderated by TaqIA A1 allele. *Science, 322*(5900), 449–452. http://dx.doi.org/10.1126/science.1161550.

Stice, E., Spoor, S., Bohon, C., Veldhuizen, M. G., & Small, D. M. (2008b). Relation of reward from food intake and anticipated food intake to obesity: A functional magnetic resonance imaging study. *Journal of Abnormal Psychology, 117*(4), 924–935. http://dx.doi.org/10.1037/a0013600.

Stoeckel, L. E., Murdaugh, D. L., Cox, J. E., Cook, E. W., 3rd., & Weller, R. E. (2013). Greater impulsivity is associated with decreased brain activation in obese women during a delay discounting task. *Brain Imaging and Behavior*, 7(2), 116–128. http://dx.doi.org/10.1007/s11682-012-9201-4.

Stojek, M. K., Fischer, S., & MacKillop, J. (2015). Stress, cues, and eating behavior. Using drug addiction paradigms to understand motivation for food. *Appetite, 92*, 252–260. http://dx.doi.org/10.1016/j.appet.2015.05.027.

Sussman, S., & Sussman, A. N. (2011). Considering the definition of addiction. *International Journal of Environmental Research and Public Health, 8*(10), 4025–4038. http://dx.doi.org/10.3390/ijerph8104025.

Tang, Y. Y., Posner, M. I., Rothbart, M. K., & Volkow, N. D. (2015). Circuitry of self-control and its role in reducing addiction. *Trends in Cognitive Sciences, 19*(8), 439–444. http://dx.doi.org/10.1016/j.tics.2015.06.007.

Tataranni, P. A., Larson, D. E., Snitker, S., Young, J. B., Flatt, J. P., & Ravussin, E. (1996). Effects of glucocorticoids on energy metabolism and food intake in humans. *The American Journal of Physiology, 271*(2 Pt. 1), E317–E325.

Taylor, S. B., Anglin, J. M., Paode, P. R., Riggert, A. G., Olive, M. F., & Conrad, C. D. (2014). Chronic stress may facilitate the recruitment of habit- and addiction-related neurocircuitries through neuronal restructuring of the striatum. *Neuroscience, 280*, 231–242. http://dx.doi.org/10.1016/j.neuroscience.2014.09.029.

The National Institute of Diabetes and Digestive and Kidney Diseases (2012). *Overweight and obesity statistics*. Retrieved from. http://www.niddk.nih.gov/health-information/health-statistics/Pages/overweight-obesity-statistics.aspx.

Thomas, J. M., Higgs, S., Dourish, C. T., Hansen, P. C., Harmer, C. J., & McCabe, C. (2015). Satiation attenuates BOLD activity in brain regions involved in reward and increases activity in dorsolateral prefrontal cortex: An fMRI study in healthy volunteers. *The American Journal of Clinical Nutrition, 101*(4), 697–704. http://dx.doi.org/10.3945/ajcn.114.097543.

Torres, S. J., & Nowson, C. A. (2007). Relationship between stress, eating behavior, and obesity. *Nutrition, 23*(11–12), 887–894. http://dx.doi.org/10.1016/j.nut.2007.08.008.

Uher, R., Murphy, T., Brammer, M. J., Dalgleish, T., Phillips, M. L., Ng, V. W., ... Treasure, J. (2004). Medial prefrontal cortex activity associated with symptom provocation in eating disorders. *The American Journal of Psychiatry*, *161*(7), 1238–1246. http://dx.doi.org/10.1176/appi.ajp.161.7.1238.

Val-Laillet, D., Aarts, E., Weber, B., Ferrari, M., Quaresima, V., Stoeckel, L. E., ... Stice, E. (2015). Neuroimaging and neuromodulation approaches to study eating behavior and prevent and treat eating disorders and obesity. *Neuroimage Clinical*, *8*, 1–31. http://dx.doi.org/10.1016/j.nicl.2015.03.016.

van Bloemendaal, L., Ten Kulve, J. S., la Fleur, S. E., Ijzerman, R. G., & Diamant, M. (2014). Effects of glucagon-like peptide 1 on appetite and body weight: Focus on the CNS. *The Journal of Endocrinology*, *221*(1), T1–T16. http://dx.doi.org/10.1530/JOE-13-0414.

van Bloemendaal, L., Veltman, D. J., Ten Kulve, J. S., Groot, P. F., Ruhe, H. G., Barkhof, F., ... Ijzerman, R. G. (2015). Brain reward-system activation in response to anticipation and consumption of palatable food is altered by glucagon-like peptide-1 receptor activation in humans. *Diabetes, Obesity & Metabolism*, *17*(9), 878–886. http://dx.doi.org/10.1111/dom.12506.

van de Giessen, E., la Fleur, S. E., Eggels, L., de Bruin, K., van den Brink, W., & Booij, J. (2013). High fat/carbohydrate ratio but not total energy intake induces lower striatal dopamine D2/3 receptor availability in diet-induced obesity. *International Journal of Obesity*, *37*(5), 754–757. http://dx.doi.org/10.1038/ijo.2012.128.

Varela, L., & Horvath, T. L. (2012). Leptin and insulin pathways in POMC and AgRP neurons that modulate energy balance and glucose homeostasis. *EMBO Reports*, *13*(12), 1079–1086. http://dx.doi.org/10.1038/embor.2012.174.

Volkow, N. D., Fowler, J. S., Wang, G. J., & Goldstein, R. Z. (2002). Role of dopamine, the frontal cortex and memory circuits in drug addiction: Insight from imaging studies. *Neurobiology of Learning and Memory*, *78*(3), 610–624.

Volkow, N. D., Wang, G. J., & Baler, R. D. (2011). Reward, dopamine and the control of food intake: Implications for obesity. *Trends in Cognitive Sciences*, *15*(1), 37–46. http://dx.doi.org/10.1016/j.tics.2010.11.001.

Volkow, N. D., Wang, G. J., Fowler, J. S., Logan, J., Gatley, S. J., Hitzemann, R., ... Pappas, N. (1997). Decreased striatal dopaminergic responsiveness in detoxified cocaine-dependent subjects. *Nature*, *386*(6627), 830–833. http://dx.doi.org/10.1038/386830a0.

Volkow, N. D., Wang, G. J., Fowler, J. S., Tomasi, D., & Baler, R. (2012). Food and drug reward: Overlapping circuits in human obesity and addiction. *Current Topics in Behavioral Neurosciences*, *11*, 1–24. http://dx.doi.org/10.1007/7854_2011_169.

Volkow, N. D., Wang, G. J., Maynard, L., Jayne, M., Fowler, J. S., Zhu, W., ... Pappas, N. (2003). Brain dopamine is associated with eating behaviors in humans. *The International Journal of Eating Disorders*, *33*(2), 136–142. http://dx.doi.org/10.1002/eat.10118.

Wang, K. S., Smith, D. V., & Delgado, M. R. (2016). Using fMRI to study reward processing in humans: Past, present, and future. *Journal of Neurophysiology*, *115*(3), 1664–1678. http://dx.doi.org/10.1152/jn.00333.2015.

Warne, J. P. (2009). Shaping the stress response: Interplay of palatable food choices, glucocorticoids, insulin and abdominal obesity. *Molecular and Cellular Endocrinology*, *300*(1–2), 137–146. http://dx.doi.org/10.1016/j.mce.2008.09.036.

Weiss, F., Ciccocioppo, R., Parsons, L. H., Katner, S., Liu, X., Zorrilla, E. P., ... Richter, R. R. (2001). Compulsive drug-seeking behavior and relapse. Neuroadaptation, stress, and conditioning factors. *Annals of the New York Academy of Sciences*, *937*, 1–26.

Wilcox, G. (2005). Insulin and insulin resistance. *Clinical Biochemist Reviews*, *26*(2), 19–39.

Winstanley, C. A., Eagle, D. M., & Robbins, T. W. (2006). Behavioral models of impulsivity in relation to ADHD: Translation between clinical and preclinical studies. *Clinical Psychology Review*, *26*(4), 379–395. http://dx.doi.org/10.1016/j.cpr.2006.01.001.

Womble, L. G., Williamson, D. A., Martin, C. K., Zucker, N. L., Thaw, J. M., Netemeyer, R., … Greenway, F. L. (2001). Psychosocial variables associated with binge eating in obese males and females. *The International Journal of Eating Disorders*, *30*(2), 217–221.

Wren, A. M., & Bloom, S. R. (2007). Gut hormones and appetite control. *Gastroenterology*, *132*(6), 2116–2130. http://dx.doi.org/10.1053/j.gastro.2007.03.048.

Ziauddeen, H., Alonso-Alonso, M., Hill, J. O., Kelley, M., & Khan, N. A. (2015). Obesity and the neurocognitive basis of food reward and the control of intake. *Advances in Nutrition*, *6*(4), 474–486. http://dx.doi.org/10.3945/an.115.008268.

Ziauddeen, H., Farooqi, I. S., & Fletcher, P. C. (2012). Obesity and the brain: How convincing is the addiction model? *Nature Reviews. Neuroscience*, *13*(4), 279–286. http://dx.doi.org/10.1038/nrn3212.

Ziauddeen, H., & Fletcher, P. C. (2013). Is food addiction a valid and useful concept? *Obesity Reviews*, *14*(1), 19–28. http://dx.doi.org/10.1111/j.1467-789X.2012.01046.x.

Zilverstand, A., Parvaz, M. A., Moeller, S. J., & Goldstein, R. Z. (2016). Cognitive interventions for addiction medicine: Understanding the underlying neurobiological mechanisms. In E. Hamed & P. P. Martin (Eds.), *Progress in brain research: Vol. 224*. (pp. 285–304). Cambridge, MA: Elsevier. chapter 13.

Zwaan, M., Engeli, S., & Muller, A. (2015). Temperamental factors in severe weight cycling. A cross-sectional study. *Appetite*, *91*, 336–342. http://dx.doi.org/10.1016/j.appet.2015.04.064.

CHAPTER FIVE

Imaging the Gambling Brain

I.M. Balodis, M.N. Potenza[1]
Yale University, New Haven, CT, United States
[1]Corresponding author: e-mail address: marc.potenza@yale.edu

Contents

Abstract

Neuroimaging studies examining the neurobiological basis of gambling disorder (GD) have increased over the past decade. Functional magnetic resonance imaging studies during appetitive cue and reward processing tasks demonstrate altered functioning in frontostriatal brain areas, including the ventral striatum and the ventromedial prefrontal cortex. Findings suggest differences in how the anticipation and outcome of rewards are processed in individuals with GD. Future research requires larger sample sizes and should include appropriate clinical reference groups. Overall, studies to date highlight a common pathophysiology between substance-based addictions and GD, the latter offering a unique condition in which to examine nonchemical factors in addiction.

The first neuroimaging study in pathological gambling (PG) was conducted in 2003 (Potenza, Steinberg, et al., 2003), since that time, neurobiological findings have demonstrated significant overlap between substance-use disorders and disordered gambling, providing substantial evidence to reclassify the disorder with other addictions. In 2013, gambling disorder (GD), formerly termed pathological gambling (PG), became the first nonsubstance-based disorder in a new "Addictions" category in the DSM-5 (APA, 2013). Over the past decade, brain imaging studies in GD have grown to over 30 directly investigating neural responses in populations with GD.

International Review of Neurobiology, Volume 129
ISSN 0074-7742
http://dx.doi.org/10.1016/bs.irn.2016.05.001

Neuroimaging studies in GD offer several unique and significant contributions to the greater addictions research field. Due to neurotoxic effects of drugs on the brain, any neural alterations in substance-based addictions can be difficult to interpret; as a "chemical-free" addiction, GD presents the prospect of examining addiction mechanisms in the brain without the confound of a drug present. Aside from the ability to disentangle contributor/consequence factors in addiction, GD neuroimaging studies provide information on decision-making processes, for example, how the brain processes probability, risk, reward, and losses. Understanding these processes has enormous implications for other research fields such as behavioral economics and even more broadly, on how people form preferences and make decisions.

1. CUE-REACTIVITY STUDIES

To date, most neuroimaging studies in GD focus on reward processing, particularly examining appetitive stimuli during cue exposure or as an individual wins various amounts of money. Examining neural responses as an individual views gambling stimuli provides information on attentional processes in GD and can offer insights into craving mechanisms for this disorder. Gambling cues, even if they are not specific to an individual's preferred gaming type, can produce cravings in a person with GD (Crockford, Goodyear, Edwards, Quickfall, & el-Guebaly, 2005). Thus cue-reactivity investigations in GD provide some insight into attentional and motivational processing, including craving in this disorder.

The first functional magnetic resonance imaging (fMRI) study in a gambling population had individuals watching gambling videos depicting various gambling situations while in the scanner (Potenza, Steinberg, et al., 2003). Results showed reduced activity in the ventromedial prefrontal cortex (vmPFC) as GD individuals, relative to healthy controls (HCs), watched the gambling situations (Potenza, Steinberg, et al., 2003). The vmPFC, located on the front, inferior portion of the brain, is reciprocally connected to many other prefrontal areas as well as the striatum, thereby making it an important region of the reward network (Ongur & Price, 2000). In particular, this brain region signals the incentive value of a stimulus and rapidly updates its activity to signal the changing value of a reinforcer (Levy & Glimcher, 2012; Noel, Brevers, & Bechara, 2013). While this early fMRI study in GD only included 10 individuals with PG, it nonetheless was the first to demonstrate neural response patterns for gambling cues that are distinct from other emotional states. Shortly thereafter, Reuter and colleagues

(2005) had participants with GD perform a guessing task and also found diminished vmPFC and reduced striatal activity relative to a control group. Reduced activity in these areas was additionally related to gambling severity: those individuals with the most severe GD showed the least striatal and vmPFC activity (Reuter et al., 2005).

Since those initial fMRI studies in GD, multiple other studies have replicated or demonstrated similar blunted frontostriatal processing in this population during cue exposure or reward processing (Balodis et al., 2012; Choi et al., 2012; de Greck et al., 2010; de Ruiter et al., 2009; Tanabe et al., 2007). These blunted reward neurocircuitry responses are similar to that seen in substance-dependent populations (Allain, Minogianis, Roberts, & Samaha, 2015), but diverge from increased frontostriatal reactivity to disorder-related cues reported in obsessive–compulsive disorder (OCD) (Saxena & Rauch, 2000). As such, fMRI studies to date provide more neurofunctional similarities in GD with substance-use disorders, than with OCD. Additionally, relationships between frontostriatal activity and measures of gambling pathology have continued to appear in the neuroimaging literature, suggesting important links between the two (eg, Balodis et al., 2012; Choi et al., 2012; de Ruiter, Oosterlaan, Veltman, van den Brink, & Goudriaan, 2012).

Nevertheless, several fMRI studies in GD demonstrate increased cortical and subcortical gambling cue reactivity. During gambling videos, Crockford and colleagues (2005) reported that a GD group showed increased activity in the dorsal visual processing stream. Specifically, individuals with GD showed greater dorsolateral prefrontal cortex activity, including the precuneus and the parahippocampal areas (Crockford et al., 2005). These brain areas are often implicated in attention, memory, and goal planning (Duncan & Owen, 2000; Gazzaley & Nobre, 2012). This early fMRI study also tested whether a relationship might exist between neural responses and physiologic reactivity; however, the investigators reported no relationship between brain activation with either respiration or heart rate.

Another study examining cue reactivity by Goudriaan, de Ruiter, van den Brink, Oosterlaan, and Veltman (2010) also found increased cortical and subcortical activity relative in a group of problem and pathological gamblers. This study included two control groups: a HC group, but also a group of heavy smokers. With two comparison groups, results demonstrated that the GD group had heightened activity when viewing gambling images in occipital, parahippocampal, amygdalar, and ventrolateral PFC areas, relative to both the heavy smokers and the HC group. While activity in some of the areas was linked to craving in the GD group, it should be noted that craving measures were not statistically significantly increased during cue exposure (Goudriaan et al., 2010). Nonetheless, this study demonstrates the ability of gambling stimuli to recruit brain areas involved in visual processing, attention, memory, and emotional processing.

One of the largest neuroimaging studies in GD was recently published, as well as one of the first specifically investigating gender differences. The study compared a GD group with a cocaine dependent (CD) and a HC group as they viewed gambling-related videos in the scanner (Kober et al., 2016). In a sample of 28 individuals with GD, investigators were able to identify differentiated neural responses in males vs females. Specifically, females with GD showed greater activity in posterior putamen/insular regions while viewing gambling-related stimuli—regions that have previously been linked to drug craving and gambling urges (Garavan, 2010; Goudriaan et al., 2010). Altogether these findings suggest important gender-related differences in motivational responses to gambling cues and that craving states may be generated differently across males and females (Kober et al., 2016). While gender differences are noted in prevalence, onset and gambling motivations, this is one of the first to directly examine sex-specific neural substrates.

2. PARSING OUT SPECIFIC COGNITIVE CONSTRUCTS IN GD

2.1 Anticipatory Processing

Technical developments and improved anatomical segmentation through neuroimaging together with conceptual refinements in GD have resulted in more specific examination of cognitive constructs. For example, several recent neuroimaging studies examine anticipatory processing in GD. Anticipation refers to the period of time immediately prior to an outcome and can comprise powerful expectancy effects. A better understanding of anticipatory processes has implications for shedding light on motivational processing, particularly those related to the construct of craving, a central addiction characteristic. In the brain, anticipatory reward processing recruits striatal neurocircuitry, whereas the receipt of reward activates more medial prefrontal cortical regions (Knutson, Adams, Fong, & Hommer, 2001; Knutson, Fong, Adams, Varner, & Hommer, 2001). Notably, craving also recruits striatal areas (Breiter, Aharon, Kahneman, Dale, & Shizgal, 2001; Knutson, Adams, et al., 2001) and relates to anticipatory processes.

One fMRI study examining anticipatory processing in a GD population found diminished frontostriatal activity relative to an HC group as they won and lost different amounts of money in the scanner (Balodis et al., 2012). Notably, activity in the ventral striatum during anticipation was inversely linked to impulsivity: the higher impulsivity score that a GD individual presented, the less activity in ventral areas of the striatum. These results show similarities to previous reports linking striatal activity with gambling severity (eg, Reuter et al., 2005). Moreover, these findings closely parallel reduced anticipatory processing in the striatum reported in an alcohol-dependent population (Beck et al., 2009) and in individuals with a family history of alcohol dependence (Andrews et al., 2011) using the same task to examine anticipatory processing. Additionally, all studies report similar inverse relationships between anticipatory striatal signaling and impulsivity. Altogether, this growing body of research suggests neurobiological similarities in the relationship between anticipatory ventral striatal signaling with the construct of impulsivity across substance-based, nonsubstance-based as well as those at risk for addiction.

Altered activity in GD has also been noted in more dorsal areas of the striatum. For example, van Holst and colleagues reported that individuals with GD demonstrate increased activity in this area when anticipating winning €5 vs €1 on a guessing paradigm (van Holst, Veltman, Buchel, van den Brink, & Goudriaan, 2012). More dorsal regions of the striatum often show increasing activity over the course of learning, as an activity becomes more habitual (Atallah, Lopez-Paniagua, Rudy, & O'Reilly, 2007; O'Doherty et al., 2004; Reading, Dunnett, & Robbins, 1991). Additionally, the dorsal striatum codes for prediction errors as well as action–outcome associations (Haruno et al., 2004; O'Doherty et al., 2004; Tricomi, Delgado, & Fiez, 2004). Thus, increased dorsal striatal activity in response to winning €5 vs €1 on a guessing paradigm might suggest *increased* sensitivity to the magnitude of reward in the GD group, and/or increased propensity to think that their actions directly influence the outcome. Further research is necessary to explore these possibilities.

2.2 Subjective Value

In addition to advances in anatomical segmentation of striatal areas, other studies are highlighting the complexity of accounting for subjective reward valuation. A study by Miedl, Peters, and Buchel (2012) examined how individuals chose between fixed immediate rewards or larger, delayed rewards.

The authors demonstrated how the ventral striatum and the vmPFC signaled the value of stimuli, additionally, however, the activation in these areas was modulated by the subjective value of the stimuli (Miedl et al., 2012). These findings demonstrate important individual difference effects on brain activity and highlight the difficulty in controlling for these factors across various paradigms and task-dependent effects as well as across diverse populations. Nevertheless, even when controlling for differences in subjective value, Miedl and colleagues still found that risky rewards produced reduced frontostriatal recruitment in the GD group relative to an HC group. Moreover, Miedl and colleagues also found an inverse relationship between frontostriatal activity during delayed rewards and problem-gambling severity. These results are once again consistent with other studies finding an inverse relationship between frontostriatal recruitment and measures of pathology (Balodis et al., 2012; Reuter et al., 2005) (Fig. 1).

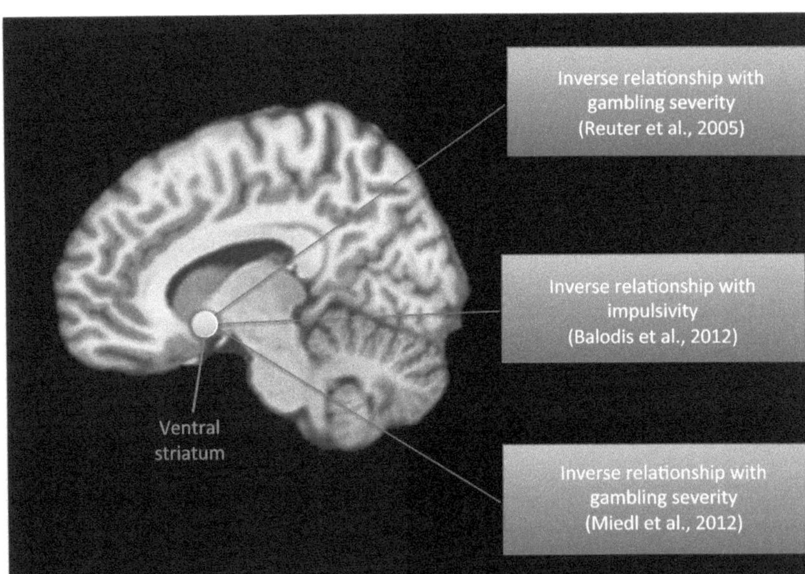

Fig. 1 Inverse relationship between striatal activity and measures of gambling pathology. Multiple neuroimaging studies demonstrate an inverse relationship between activity in frontostriatal areas and measures of gambling pathology, particularly in striatal areas. *Blue* (*white in the print version*) *circle* highlights the ventral striatum ($x=9$).

2.3 Near Misses

"Near misses" are a unique feature of gambling that can have a profound effect on the individual. Several GD studies have examined the "near miss" phenomena, whereby a loss is perceived as almost winning. These near miss effects, while subjectively producing unpleasant feelings, nonetheless activate reward neurocircuitry and effectively increase the motivation to gamble (Chase & Clark, 2010; Clark et al., 2012; Worhunsky, Malison, Rogers, & Potenza, 2014). One recent neuroimaging study examining this effect compared a GD group with a HC as well as a CD group as they played a slot-machine task in the scanner (Worhunsky et al., 2014). Results showed that both the GD and the CD groups had amplified anticipatory responding in reward neurocircuitry to a near miss event. These findings can therefore provide a mechanistic idea of how near misses still stimulate reward neurocircuitry and generate cognitive distortions about control and winning thereby encouraging continued playing. In regular gamblers, near miss events produce increased activity in dopamine-rich areas, which further relates to gambling severity (Chase & Clark, 2010; Clark, Lawrence, Astley-Jones, & Gray, 2009).

Recently, neuroimaging studies examine not only brain areas activated by gambling stimuli but also how these areas communicate with each other. One neuroimaging study used functional connectivity to investigate near miss events across a population of regular and nonregular gamblers (van Holst, Chase, & Clark, 2014). The investigators reported stronger striatal–insula connections were related to greater illusions of control. These findings suggest that increased connections between reward circuitry and areas involved in interoceptive processing may lead to distorted beliefs about winning and ultimately promote loss-chasing in some individuals. Further research into understanding the neural mechanisms underlying cognitive distortions will be important.

2.4 Inhibitory Control Studies

To date, only a handful of imaging studies have examined inhibitory processing in GD. One early study of cognitive control had participants perform the Stroop task while undergoing fMRI (Potenza, Leung, et al., 2003). The Stroop task is a cognitive control task in which individuals name the color of a word, rather than read the word. This requires a person to inhibit the prepotent response of reading and effectively recruits inhibitory neurocircuitry including the anterior cingulate and dorsolateral prefrontal cortex when the color of the word is incongruent with the word meaning (eg, the word "red" written in green ink). In a GD population, incongruent trials produce reduced vmPFC activity in a GD population relative to an HC group (Potenza, Leung, et al., 2003). Another task examining inhibition is the Stop Signal Task, which has the advantage of examining the neural substrates of error processing and response suppression once an action has been initiated. An elegant study by de Ruiter and colleagues found that during successful inhibition, relative to an HC group, GD individuals demonstrated reduced activity in dorsomedial prefrontal and anterior cingulate areas (de Ruiter et al., 2012). Additionally, activity in this latter area was inversely related to gambling severity, demonstrating that problem-gambling severity relates to recruitment of inhibitory neurocircuitry. Another well-designed feature of this study was the inclusion of a heavy smoker group who further demonstrated diminished processing in overlapping dorsomedial prefrontal and cingulate areas. Thus, heavy smokers and individuals with GD display hypoactivations in inhibitory neurocircuitry during inhibition, thereby providing additional support for similar neurobiological alterations across substance- and nonsubstance-based disorders.

3. POSITRON EMISSION TOMOGRAPHY STUDIES

A growing number of GD studies are also applying positron emission tomography (PET) scans to examine specific neurotransmitter systems potentially underlying dysregulated behavior. To date, most investigations have focused on dopamine, given its role in reward processing, substance dependence and the striatum as a key projection area for this neurotransmitter. Additionally, findings from a disorder characterized by reduced dopamine availability, Parkinson's Disease, provided some indications for dopamine's role in impulsive behaviors. Multiple studies now document the development of gambling problems and other impulse control problems, following dopamine replacement therapies in Parkinson's (Leeman & Potenza, 2011; Molina et al., 2000). Following administration of drugs that increase brain dopamine levels, some individuals with Parkinson's disease have developed problem behaviors, including gambling, sex, and shopping (Weintraub & Potenza, 2006; Weintraub et al., 2010). Nonetheless findings from PET imaging in GD have had complicated and mixed results. For example, one study examining dopamine changes as individuals performed the Iowa Gambling Task (IGT) did not find that all participants showed dopamine increases in conjunction with the task (Linnet, Moller, Peterson, Gjedde, & Doudet, 2011). However, those individuals with GD who did show increased dopamine release were also those who reported greater excitement levels, although their performance was significantly poorer on the IGT. Thus the relationship between gambling excitement and dopamine release remains unclear, suggesting additional contributors. To date, several PET studies have not detected differences in the D2-like receptors when comparing GD with HC populations (Boileau et al., 2013; Joutsa et al., 2012), leading some to question the centrality of dopamine in GD (Potenza, 2013).

Following an amphetamine challenge, a recent PET study reported that individuals with GD had increased dopamine release in the striatum (Boileau et al., 2014). These findings are in contrast to PET studies in substance dependence, which report *reduced* dopamine release following drug challenges (Martinez et al., 2005).

Nonetheless, several PET studies describe relationships between dopamine availability and impulsivity or gambling-related measures (Boileau et al., 2014; Clark et al., 2012; Joutsa et al., 2012).

Altogether, the discrepant findings suggest that dopamine may differentially contribute to addiction symptoms in GD and/or may not play as central a role in this disorder (Potenza, 2013). Future studies including larger samples, as well as directly comparing clinical reference groups will be important in clarifying the role of this neurotransmitter in GD.

4. STRUCTURAL IMAGING

Recently, the first few structural imaging studies have emerged in GD, however, most do not find gray matter differences (Joutsa et al., 2012; Koehler et al., 2013; van Holst, de Ruiter, van den Brink, Veltman, & Goudriaan, 2012). One study found that a GD group had intermediary gray matter levels between an alcohol-dependent and an HC group, suggestive that the lower gray matter levels detected in alcohol dependence may represent a neurotoxic result of chronic alcohol use (van Holst, de Ruiter, et al., 2012). Nonetheless, another recent study controlling for comorbid conditions found reduced hippocampal and amygdalar relative to an HC group (Rahman, Xu, & Potenza, 2014). Some recent studies have detected white matter alterations in limbic and prefrontal regions that may suggest a first phase of neuropathology, prior to larger regional volume changes (Joutsa et al., 2012; Yip et al., 2013). More functional connectivity studies are necessary to evaluate these networks and their relationship with functional alterations.

5. CONCLUSIONS

Neuroimaging studies in GD are becoming more numerous and are contributing to our knowledge of the pathophysiology of addiction. These studies hold much potential in untangling some of the cause and consequence effects of addiction and probing aberrant learning mechanisms in the brain. However, until recently, most neuroimaging studies in GD have included very small samples; therefore, larger studies and replications are still necessary in order to move the field forward. Longitudinal studies and subgrouping will also be crucial in shedding light on the neuropsychology and neurobiology of GD.

Nonetheless, investigators are beginning to combine methodologies across neuroimaging, genetic, psychopharmacology, and cognitive fields. For example, one pilot study found that individuals with differences in a specific gene that breaks down dopamine in the prefrontal cortex responded better to a drug enhancing dopamine activity (Grant et al., 2013)—improvements were additionally related to increased frontal activity during an executive planning task (Grant et al., 2013). Thus, these studies are beginning to identify subgroups that might best respond to a specific treatment and can further pinpoint the mechanisms by which it may be working. Larger studies are still needed; nonetheless, these findings hold promise for more targeted interventions in the future. To date, neuroimaging studies demonstrate common pathophysiology between substance-based disorders and GD. Nonetheless these studies also highlight the heterogeneity of GD and the complexity of exploring how the brain makes decisions.

REFERENCES

Allain, F., Minogianis, E. A., Roberts, D. C., & Samaha, A. N. (2015). How fast and how often: The pharmacokinetics of drug use are decisive in addiction. *Neuroscience and Biobehavioral Reviews*, *56*, 166–179. http://dx.doi.org/10.1016/j.neubiorev.2015.06.012.

Andrews, M. M., Meda, S. A., Thomas, A. D., Potenza, M. N., Krystal, J. H., Worhunsky, P., … Pearlson, G. D. (2011). Individuals family history positive for alcoholism show functional magnetic resonance imaging differences in reward sensitivity that are related to impulsivity factors. *Biological Psychiatry*, *69*(7), 675–683. http://dx.doi.org/10.1016/j.biopsych.2010.09.049. S0006-3223(10)01018-8 [pii].

APA. (2013). *Diagnostic and statistical manual of mental disorders* (5th ed.). Washington, DC: American Psychiatric Association.

Atallah, H. E., Lopez-Paniagua, D., Rudy, J. W., & O'Reilly, R. C. (2007). Separate neural substrates for skill learning and performance in the ventral and dorsal striatum. *Nature Neuroscience*, *10*(1), 126–131. http://dx.doi.org/10.1038/nn1817. nn1817 [pii].

Balodis, I. M., Kober, H., Worhunsky, P. D., Stevens, M. C., Pearlson, G. D., & Potenza, M. N. (2012). Diminished frontostriatal activity during processing of monetary rewards and losses in pathological gambling. *Biological Psychiatry*, *71*(8), 749–757. http://dx.doi.org/10.1016/j.biopsych.2012.01.006. S0006-3223(12)00044-3 [pii].

Beck, A., Schlagenhauf, F., Wustenberg, T., Hein, J., Kienast, T., Kahnt, T., ... Wrase, J. (2009). Ventral striatal activation during reward anticipation correlates with impulsivity in alcoholics. *Biological Psychiatry*, *66*(8), 734–742. http://dx.doi.org/10.1016/j.biopsych.2009.04.035. S0006-3223(09)00567-8 [pii].

Boileau, I., Payer, D., Chugani, B., Lobo, D., Behzadi, A., Rusjan, P. M., ... Zack, M. (2013). The D2/3 dopamine receptor in pathological gambling: A positron emission tomography study with [11C]-(+)-propyl-hexahydro-naphtho-oxazin and [11C] raclopride. *Addiction*, *108*(5), 953–963. http://dx.doi.org/10.1111/add.12066.

Boileau, I., Payer, D., Chugani, B., Lobo, D. S., Houle, S., Wilson, A. A., ... Zack, M. (2014). In vivo evidence for greater amphetamine-induced dopamine release in pathological gambling: A positron emission tomography study with [(11)C]-(+)-PHNO. *Molecular Psychiatry*, *19*(12), 1305–1313. http://dx.doi.org/10.1038/mp.2013.163.

Breiter, H. C., Aharon, I., Kahneman, D., Dale, A., & Shizgal, P. (2001). Functional imaging of neural responses to expectancy and experience of monetary gains and losses. *Neuron*, *30*(2), 619–639. S0896-6273(01)00303-8 [pii].

Chase, H. W., & Clark, L. (2010). Gambling severity predicts midbrain response to near-miss outcomes. *The Journal of Neuroscience*, *30*(18), 6180–6187. http://dx.doi.org/10.1523/JNEUROSCI.5758-09.2010.

Choi, J. S., Shin, Y. C., Jung, W. H., Jang, J. H., Kang, D. H., Choi, C. H., ... Kwon, J. S. (2012). Altered brain activity during reward anticipation in pathological gambling and obsessive-compulsive disorder. *PLoS One*. 7(9). e45938, http://dx.doi.org/10.1371/journal.pone.0045938. PONE-D-12-13663 [pii].

Clark, L., Lawrence, A. J., Astley-Jones, F., & Gray, N. (2009). Gambling near-misses enhance motivation to gamble and recruit win-related brain circuitry. *Neuron*, *61*(3), 481–490. http://dx.doi.org/10.1016/j.neuron.2008.12.031.

Clark, L., Stokes, P. R., Wu, K., Michalczuk, R., Benecke, A., Watson, B. J., ... Lingford-Hughes, A. R. (2012). Striatal dopamine D(2)/D(3) receptor binding in pathological gambling is correlated with mood-related impulsivity. *NeuroImage*, *63*(1), 40–46. http://dx.doi.org/10.1016/j.neuroimage.2012.06.067.

Crockford, D. N., Goodyear, B., Edwards, J., Quickfall, J., & el-Guebaly, N. (2005). Cue-induced brain activity in pathological gamblers. *Biological Psychiatry*, *58*(10), 787–795. http://dx.doi.org/10.1016/j.biopsych.2005.04.037. S0006-3223(05)00498-1 [pii].

de Greck, M., Enzi, B., Prosch, U., Gantman, A., Tempelmann, C., & Northoff, G. (2010). Decreased neuronal activity in reward circuitry of pathological gamblers during processing of personal relevant stimuli. *Human Brain Mapping*, *31*(11), 1802–1812. http://dx.doi.org/10.1002/hbm.20981.

de Ruiter, M. B., Oosterlaan, J., Veltman, D. J., van den Brink, W., & Goudriaan, A. E. (2012). Similar hyporesponsiveness of the dorsomedial prefrontal cortex in problem gamblers and heavy smokers during an inhibitory control task. *Drug and Alcohol Dependence*, *121*(1–2), 81–89. http://dx.doi.org/10.1016/j.drugalcdep.2011.08.010.

de Ruiter, M. B., Veltman, D. J., Goudriaan, A. E., Oosterlaan, J., Sjoerds, Z., & van den Brink, W. (2009). Response perseveration and ventral prefrontal sensitivity to reward and punishment in male problem gamblers and smokers. *Neuropsychopharmacology*, *34*(4), 1027–1038. http://dx.doi.org/10.1038/npp.2008.175.

Duncan, J., & Owen, A. M. (2000). Common regions of the human frontal lobe recruited by diverse cognitive demands. *Trends in Neurosciences*, *23*(10), 475–483.

Garavan, H. (2010). Insula and drug cravings. *Brain Structure & Function*, *214*(5–6), 593–601. http://dx.doi.org/10.1007/s00429-010-0259-8.

Gazzaley, A., & Nobre, A. C. (2012). Top-down modulation: Bridging selective attention and working memory. *Trends in Cognitive Sciences*, *16*(2), 129–135. http://dx.doi.org/10.1016/j.tics.2011.11.014.

Goudriaan, A. E., de Ruiter, M. B., van den Brink, W., Oosterlaan, J., & Veltman, D. J. (2010). Brain activation patterns associated with cue reactivity and craving in abstinent problem gamblers, heavy smokers and healthy controls: An fMRI study. *Addiction Biology*, *15*(4), 491–503. http://dx.doi.org/10.1111/j.1369-1600.2010.00242.x.

Grant, J. E., Odlaug, B. L., Chamberlain, S. R., Hampshire, A., Schreiber, L. R., & Kim, S. W. (2013). A proof of concept study of tolcapone for pathological gambling: Relationships with COMT genotype and brain activation. *European Neuropsychopharmacology*, *23*(11), 1587–1596. http://dx.doi.org/10.1016/j.euroneuro.2013.07.008.

Haruno, M., Kuroda, T., Doya, K., Toyama, K., Kimura, M., Samejima, K., … Kawato, M. (2004). A neural correlate of reward-based behavioral learning in caudate nucleus: A functional magnetic resonance imaging study of a stochastic decision task. *The Journal of Neuroscience*, *24*(7), 1660–1665. http://dx.doi.org/10.1523/JNEUROSCI.3417-03.2004. 24/7/1660 [pii].

Joutsa, J., Johansson, J., Niemela, S., Ollikainen, A., Hirvonen, M. M., Piepponen, P., … Kaasinen, V. (2012). Mesolimbic dopamine release is linked to symptom severity in pathological gambling. *NeuroImage*, *60*(4), 1992–1999. http://dx.doi.org/10.1016/j.neuroimage.2012.02.006.

Knutson, B., Adams, C. M., Fong, G. W., & Hommer, D. (2001). Anticipation of increasing monetary reward selectively recruits nucleus accumbens. *The Journal of Neuroscience*, *21*(16), RC159. 20015472 [pii].

Knutson, B., Fong, G. W., Adams, C. M., Varner, J. L., & Hommer, D. (2001). Dissociation of reward anticipation and outcome with event-related fMRI. *Neuroreport*, *12*(17), 3683–3687.

Kober, H., Lacadie, C. M., Wexler, B. E., Malison, R. T., Sinha, R., & Potenza, M. N. (2016). Brain activity during cocaine craving and gambling urges: An fMRI study. *Neuropsychopharmacology*, *41*(2), 628–637. http://dx.doi.org/10.1038/npp.2015.193.

Koehler, S., Ovadia-Caro, S., van der Meer, E., Villringer, A., Heinz, A., Romanczuk-Seiferth, N., & Margulies, D. S. (2013). Increased functional connectivity between prefrontal cortex and reward system in pathological gambling. *PLoS One*, *8*(12). e84565, http://dx.doi.org/10.1371/journal.pone.0084565.

Leeman, R. F., & Potenza, M. N. (2011). Impulse control disorders in Parkinson's disease: Clinical characteristics and implications. *Neuropsychiatry*, *1*(2), 133–147. http://dx.doi.org/10.2217/npy.11.11.

Levy, D. J., & Glimcher, P. W. (2012). The root of all value: A neural common currency for choice. *Current Opinion in Neurobiology*, *22*(6), 1027–1038. http://dx.doi.org/10.1016/j.conb.2012.06.001.

Linnet, J., Moller, A., Peterson, E., Gjedde, A., & Doudet, D. (2011). Dopamine release in ventral striatum during Iowa Gambling Task performance is associated with increased excitement levels in pathological gambling. *Addiction*, *106*(2), 383–390. http://dx.doi.org/10.1111/j.1360-0443.2010.03126.x.

Martinez, D., Gil, R., Slifstein, M., Hwang, D. R., Huang, Y., Perez, A., … Abi-Dargham, A. (2005). Alcohol dependence is associated with blunted dopamine transmission in the ventral striatum. *Biological Psychiatry*, *58*(10), 779–786. http://dx.doi.org/10.1016/j.biopsych.2005.04.044.

Miedl, S. F., Peters, J., & Buchel, C. (2012). Altered neural reward representations in pathological gamblers revealed by delay and probability discounting. *Archives of General Psychiatry*, *69*(2), 177–186. http://dx.doi.org/10.1001/archgenpsychiatry.2011.1552.

Molina, J. A., Sainz-Artiga, M. J., Fraile, A., Jimenez-Jimenez, F. J., Villanueva, C., Orti-Pareja, M., & Bermejo, F. (2000). Pathologic gambling in Parkinson's disease:

A behavioral manifestation of pharmacologic treatment? *Movement Disorders*, *15*(5), 869–872.

Noel, X., Brevers, D., & Bechara, A. (2013). A neurocognitive approach to understanding the neurobiology of addiction. *Current Opinion in Neurobiology*, *23*(4), 632–638. http://dx.doi.org/10.1016/j.conb.2013.01.018.

O'Doherty, J., Dayan, P., Schultz, J., Deichmann, R., Friston, K., & Dolan, R. J. (2004). Dissociable roles of ventral and dorsal striatum in instrumental conditioning. *Science*, *304*(5669), 452–454. http://dx.doi.org/10.1126/science.1094285. 304/5669/452 [pii].

Ongur, D., & Price, J. L. (2000). The organization of networks within the orbital and medial prefrontal cortex of rats, monkeys and humans. *Cerebral Cortex*, *10*(3), 206–219.

Potenza, M. N. (2013). How central is dopamine to pathological gambling or gambling disorder? *Frontiers in Behavioral Neuroscience*, 7, 206. http://dx.doi.org/10.3389/fnbeh.2013.00206.

Potenza, M. N., Leung, H. C., Blumberg, H. P., Peterson, B. S., Fulbright, R. K., Lacadie, C. M., … Gore, J. C. (2003). An FMRI Stroop task study of ventromedial prefrontal cortical function in pathological gamblers. *The American Journal of Psychiatry*, *160*(11), 1990–1994.

Potenza, M. N., Steinberg, M. A., Skudlarski, P., Fulbright, R. K., Lacadie, C. M., Wilber, M. K., … Wexler, B. E. (2003). Gambling urges in pathological gambling: A functional magnetic resonance imaging study. *Archives of General Psychiatry*, *60*(8), 828–836. http://dx.doi.org/10.1001/archpsyc.60.8.828. 60/8/828 [pii].

Rahman, A. S., Xu, J., & Potenza, M. N. (2014). Hippocampal and amygdalar volumetric differences in pathological gambling: A preliminary study of the associations with the behavioral inhibition system. *Neuropsychopharmacology*, *39*(3), 738–745. http://dx.doi.org/10.1038/npp.2013.260.

Reading, P. J., Dunnett, S. B., & Robbins, T. W. (1991). Dissociable roles of the ventral, medial and lateral striatum on the acquisition and performance of a complex visual stimulus-response habit. *Behavioural Brain Research*, *45*(2), 147–161.

Reuter, J., Raedler, T., Rose, M., Hand, I., Glascher, J., & Buchel, C. (2005). Pathological gambling is linked to reduced activation of the mesolimbic reward system. *Nature Neuroscience*, *8*(2), 147–148. http://dx.doi.org/10.1038/nn1378. nn1378 [pii].

Saxena, S., & Rauch, S. L. (2000). Functional neuroimaging and the neuroanatomy of obsessive-compulsive disorder. *The Psychiatric Clinics of North America*, *23*(3), 563–586.

Tanabe, J., Thompson, L., Claus, E., Dalwani, M., Hutchison, K., & Banich, M. T. (2007). Prefrontal cortex activity is reduced in gambling and nongambling substance users during decision-making. *Human Brain Mapping*, *28*(12), 1276–1286. http://dx.doi.org/10.1002/hbm.20344.

Tricomi, E. M., Delgado, M. R., & Fiez, J. A. (2004). Modulation of caudate activity by action contingency. *Neuron*, *41*(2), 281–292. S0896627303008481 [pii].

van Holst, R. J., Chase, H. W., & Clark, L. (2014). Striatal connectivity changes following gambling wins and near-misses: Associations with gambling severity. *NeuroImage. Clinical*, *5*, 232–239. http://dx.doi.org/10.1016/j.nicl.2014.06.008.

van Holst, R. J., de Ruiter, M. B., van den Brink, W., Veltman, D. J., & Goudriaan, A. E. (2012). A voxel-based morphometry study comparing problem gamblers, alcohol abusers, and healthy controls. *Drug and Alcohol Dependence*, *124*(1–2), 142–148. http://dx.doi.org/10.1016/j.drugalcdep.2011.12.025.

van Holst, R. J., Veltman, D. J., Buchel, C., van den Brink, W., & Goudriaan, A. E. (2012). Distorted expectancy coding in problem gambling: Is the addictive in the anticipation? *Biological Psychiatry*, *71*(8), 741–748. http://dx.doi.org/10.1016/j.biopsych.2011.12.030.

Weintraub, D., Koester, J., Potenza, M. N., Siderowf, A. D., Stacy, M., Voon, V., … Lang, A. E. (2010). Impulse control disorders in Parkinson disease: A cross-sectional

study of 3090 patients. *Archives of Neurology*, *67*(5), 589–595. http://dx.doi.org/10.1001/archneurol.2010.65.
Weintraub, D., & Potenza, M. N. (2006). Impulse control disorders in Parkinson's disease. *Current Neurology and Neuroscience Reports*, *6*(4), 302–306.
Worhunsky, P. D., Malison, R. T., Rogers, R. D., & Potenza, M. N. (2014). Altered neural correlates of reward and loss processing during simulated slot-machine fMRI in pathological gambling and cocaine dependence. *Drug and Alcohol Dependence*, *145*, 77–86. http://dx.doi.org/10.1016/j.drugalcdep.2014.09.013.
Yip, S. W., Lacadie, C., Xu, J., Worhunsky, P. D., Fulbright, R. K., Constable, R. T., & Potenza, M. N. (2013). Reduced genual corpus callosal white matter integrity in pathological gambling and its relationship to alcohol abuse or dependence. *The World Journal of Biological Psychiatry*, *14*(2), 129–138. http://dx.doi.org/10.3109/15622975.2011.568068.

CHAPTER SIX

Biomarkers for Success: Using Neuroimaging to Predict Relapse and Develop Brain Stimulation Treatments for Cocaine-Dependent Individuals

C.A. Hanlon[1], L.T. Dowdle, J.L. Jones
Medical University of South Carolina, Charleston, SC, United States
[1]Corresponding author: e-mail address: hanlon@musc.edu

Contents

Abstract

Cocaine dependence is one of the most difficult substance use disorders to treat. While the powerful effects of cocaine use on behavior were documented in the 19th century, it was not until the late 20th century that we realized cocaine use was affecting brain tissue and function. Following a brief introduction (Section 1), this chapter will summarize our current knowledge regarding alterations in neural circuit function typically observed in chronic cocaine users (Section 2) and highlight an emerging body of literature which suggests that pretreatment limbic circuit activity may be a reliable predictor of clinical outcomes among individuals seeking treatment for cocaine (Section 3). Finally, as the field of addiction research strives to translate this neuroimaging data into

International Review of Neurobiology, Volume 129
ISSN 0074-7742
http://dx.doi.org/10.1016/bs.irn.2016.06.006

something clinically meaningful, we will highlight several new brain stimulation approaches which utilize functional brain imaging data to design noninvasive brain stimulation interventions for individuals seeking treatment for substance dependence disorders (Section 4).

1. INTRODUCTION

Dr. Watson, admiring Sherlock Holmes, "But consider!...Count the cost! Your brain may, as you say, be roused and excited, but it is a pathological and morbid process which involves increased tissue change and may at least leave permanent weakness....Why should you, for a mere passing pleasure, risk the loss of those great powers with which you have been endowed?"

Sign of Four, Sherlock Holmes (Doyle, 1890)

This quote from Dr. Watson comes as a plea to Sherlock Holmes who has taken up the bad habit of using cocaine in a "seven-per-cent solution" when he is feeling bored. Whether Sir Arthur Conan Doyle realized it or not this may be one of the first suggestions that regular use of cocaine could change the structure of the brain. Over 100 years later, the recreational use of cocaine, which was present in Sir Arthur Conan Doyle's time, has evolved to become a massive public health concern. In the 2013 National Survey of Drug Use and Health, approximately 1.5 million people used cocaine in the previous month (2014). The overall costs associated with cocaine and other illicit drug use was estimated at $180 billion, with an annual rate of increase of 5.34% over the preceding decade. In addition to causing psychosocial and economic hardship on the dependent individuals and their families, chronic cocaine use also leads to higher rates of myocardial infarction, arrhythmias, heart failure, stroke, rhabdomyolysis, intestinal ischemia, aortic dissection, seizures, bronchospasm, pulmonary edema, hypertensive emergency, and bruxism (sometimes leading to severe dental damage), as well as exposure to infectious diseases such as HIV and hepatitis (Afonso, Mohammad, & Thatai, 2007; Boghdadi & Henning, 1997; Pallasch & Joseph, 1987; Tseng, Sutter, & Albertson, 2014).

After the surge of cocaine use that occurred in the United States in the 1980s, Congress dubbed the subsequent years the "Decade of the Brain." At this point, scientific research regarding the effects of chronic cocaine use on the brain grew exponentially. The fictional assertion from 221 Baker Street regarding cocaine's effects on the brain can now be supported by shelves of brain imaging journals in the nonfiction section of your local university. Through structural magnetic resonance imaging (MRI), we now know that chronic cocaine use is associated with a loss of gray matter. Through diffusion tensor imaging, we have found that this gray matter disruption is accompanied by white matter decay. Positron emission tomography (PET) imaging has reliably demonstrated that acute cocaine exposure leads to a change in dopamine binding in the striatum, and that chronic exposure leads to a cascade of changes in dopamine binding which extend from the ventral, reward-based areas of the brain to dorsal, habit-based areas. These data have also been supported by nonhuman primate studies of acute and chronic cocaine use (Hanlon, Beveridge, & Porrino, 2013).

We also now know that the neuropathology present in cocaine-dependent individuals is not restricted to a single brain region, a single-cell type, or a single neurotransmitter system. Through advances in functional neuroimaging, it is apparent that there is a distinct temporal progression many individuals experience with cocaine use; this begins with initial exposure and can progress to dependence, abstinence, and unfortunately often to relapse. This progression involves neural dysregulation in several fronto-striatal systems which contribute to behavior, notably executive function (often thought of as cognition) and limbic system processing. These systems span both cortical and subcortical regions of the brain, and they are vulnerable to pathology not only in a local population of cells but also in the white matter tracts that connect these regions. Through functional MRI (fMRI), we are now able to investigate alterations in neural circuits that are present at baseline (ie, before treatment) in chronic cocaine users, as well as alterations that occur when treatment-seeking individuals are exposed to cocaine cues or engaged in a cognitive control task.

The initial goal of this chapter is to more thoroughly describe the aberrant functionality of the executive-control and limbic-arousal neural circuits that are often implicated in addiction (Section 2). We will then further review the recent evidence which suggests that some of these circuits may be useful predictors of relapse in treatment-engaged individuals (Section 3). Finally, we will describe the initial efforts to use this knowledge of the pathologic neurocircuitry to improve patient care and deliver more effective treatments to cocaine-addicted individuals (Section 4).

2. EXECUTIVE AND LIMBIC SYSTEM ABNORMALITIES IN COCAINE-DEPENDENT INDIVIDUALS

The basic mechanism through which acute cocaine acts on the brain is through blockade of the dopamine transporter protein; this increases the duration that dopamine remains in the synaptic cleft and is able to activate the dopaminergic postsynaptic neurons. There are four principle dopaminergic pathways in the brain: the mesolimbic, mesocortical, nigrostriatal, and tuberoinfundibular circuits. Of these, the mesolimbic circuit (connecting the ventral tegmental area to the nucleus accumbens) and mesocortical circuit (connecting the ventral tegmental area to the cerebral cortex) have been the primary focus of addiction science (Fig. 1). Both of

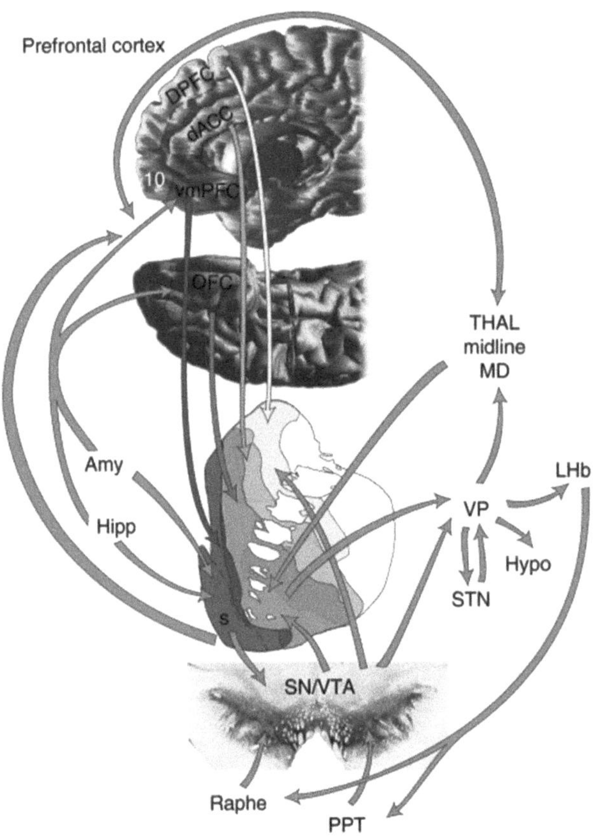

Fig. 1 Illustration of the structural connectivity between various prefrontal cortical areas to various dorsal and ventral striatal areas. The other major inputs and outputs of the striatum are also shown. *Amy*, amygdala; *BNST*, bed nucleus of the stria terminalis; *dACC*, dorsal anterior cingulate cortex; *DPFC*, dorsolateral prefrontal cortex; *Hipp*, hippocampus; *Hypo*, hypothalamus; *OFC*, orbitofrontal cortex; *PPT*, pedunculopontine nucleus; *Thal/MD*, medio-dorsal nucleus of the thalamus; *vmPFC*, ventromediąl prefrontal cortex; *VP*, ventral pallidum; *VTA/STN*, ventral tegmental area, subthalamic nucleus. *From Haber, S. N., & Knutson, B. (2010). The reward circuit: Linking primate anatomy and human imaging.* Neuropsychopharmacology, *35(1), 4–26. doi: 10.1038/npp.2009.129.*

these circuits are involved in the modulation of cognitive control, impulsivity, and habit formation experienced by cocaine users (Goldstein & Volkow, 2002). They mediate the initial volitional (and reward-based) nature of cocaine use, which eventually becomes an automatic response (ie, a habit). Animal studies have demonstrated that the mesolimbic dopamine system regulates the rewarding, reinforcing properties of cocaine. As recreational drug use progresses to addiction, the rewarding properties of the drug become less salient, and drug taking becomes guided by conditioned responses and habit; these compulsive behaviors are mediated by the *mesocortical* system (Everitt & Robbins, 2005; Porrino, Lyons, Smith, Daunais, & Nader, 2004). As such, chronic cocaine use affects not only the subcortical limbic (reward-based) circuitry but also the cortical structures that are involved in executive function (eg, attention, planning, and decision making).

2.1 Abnormalities in the Structure and Function of the Cerebral Cortex

There is broad evidence of decreased prefrontal cortex activity across multiple imaging modalities, including measures of glucose metabolism (Volkow et al., 1991), dopamine binding (Volkow et al., 1993), and blood-oxygen level-dependent (BOLD) activity, as well as measures of neural integrity (Fein, Di Sclafani, & Meyerhoff, 2002; Franklin et al., 2002; O'Neill, Cardenas, & Meyerhoff, 2001). Within the cerebral cortex, the medial prefrontal cortex (mPFC), the orbitofrontal cortex (OFC), and the dorsolateral prefrontal cortex (DLPFC) have been most extensively studied in cocaine addiction.

2.1.1 Medial Prefrontal Cortex

The mPFC extends throughout the medial section of the frontal cortex and into the OFC (BA 10). Gray matter volume in the mPFC is lower in cocaine users than in nonusers (Ersche et al., 2011; Matochik, London, Eldreth, Cadet, & Bolla, 2003). Additionally, structural imaging studies in cocaine users and abstainers have revealed that longer duration of cocaine use is associated with decreased mPFC gray matter volume (Ide et al., 2014) and that individuals abstinent from cocaine for 6 months have larger mPFC and OFC gray matter volumes compared to their actively drug-using counterparts (Hanlon, Dufault, Wesley, & Porrino, 2011). Furthermore, extended abstinence (approximately 36 weeks) may lead to recovery in volume of frontal cortical gray matter regions (Connolly, Bell, Foxe, & Garavan, 2013).

Recent longitudinal work supports these findings, showing increases in prefrontal gray matter volume over 6 months of abstinence (Parvaz et al., 2016). Functional studies using PET and fMRI have also shown that cocaine users have higher activity in mPFC when exposed to cocaine cues as opposed to neutral cues (Garavan et al., 2000; Grant et al., 1996). In contrast to the ventral aspects of the mPFC which are typically thought to be involved in mediating limbic arousal, dorsal aspects of the mPFC appear to contribute to the cognitive decrements seen in cocaine users. Evidence for this is found in functional imaging studies that show hypoactivation in the dorsal mPFC during executive function tasks among cocaine users compared to nonusers (Bolla et al., 2003; Kaufman, Ross, Stein, & Garavan, 2003; Kubler, Murphy, & Garavan, 2005). Moreover, the hypoactivation of the mPFC during an executive function task of selective attention (eg, the Stroop task) was associated with faster cocaine relapse rates (Brewer, Worhunsky, Carroll, Rounsaville, & Potenza, 2008).

2.1.2 Orbitofrontal Cortex

The OFC is located on the ventral aspect of the PFC and may contribute to the reinforcing properties of cocaine by acting as an information integrator. From a structural imaging perspective, individuals that chronically use cocaine have decreased gray matter volume in the OFC compared to nonusing controls (Matochik et al., 2003); furthermore, this volume deficit has been linked with longer duration and compulsive cocaine use (Ersche et al., 2011; Franklin et al., 2002; Sim et al., 2007). From a functional perspective, acute cocaine intoxication correlates with increased activity in the OFC and decreased activity during protracted withdrawal (Volkow & Fowler, 2000). Functional neuroimaging has also shown higher activation of the OFC during self-reported craving; the OFC is active in response to both implicit and explicit cocaine cues (Bonson et al., 2002; Childress et al., 2008). Among abstinent cocaine users, hypoactivity in the OFC during a reward-related task was linked with increased amount of drug use prior to abstinence (Bolla et al., 2003). The OFC has also been implicated in response to inhibition and this dysregulation may contribute to the continued use of cocaine despite the loss of the euphoric "high" which is seen with chronic use. Disruption of the OFC has been associated with risky decision making and an inability to anticipate outcomes (Krawczyk, 2002). Furthermore, it has been associated with perceiving the value of a stimulus, such as reward, and in learning the association between a stimulus and outcome (Kringelbach & Rolls, 2004).

2.1.3 Dorsolateral Prefrontal Cortex

The DLPFC sends afferent projections to the dorsal striatum (ie, the caudate and the putamen) and is involved in higher order processes, such as conscious decision making, reasoning, working memory, inhibition, as well as outcome prediction (Krawczyk, 2002). Structural imaging suggests that cocaine users have a significant reduction in cortical thickness in the DLPFC compared to controls (Makris et al., 2008). In a PET study, abstinent cocaine users were found to have less activation in the DLPFC when engaging in reward-related, decision-making tasks compared to nonusers (Bolla et al., 2003). However, less BOLD signal in the DLPFC during a task of attention in cocaine users prior to entering treatment predicted longer stays in treatment; this suggests that decreased utilization of the DLPFC during this task may be associated with more efficient processing and greater decision-making abilities (Brewer et al., 2008).

2.2 Abnormalities in the Structure and Function of the Subcortical Structures

2.2.1 Nucleus Accumbens

The nucleus accumbens (NAcc) is a small structure located in the ventral striatum. From a clinical neuroimaging perspective, the NAcc is difficult to image given its size and proximity to cerebral sinuses and pulsating arterioles. Specifically, the NAcc is approximately 1–2 cm^3 in humans relative to a whole-brain volume of 1100+ cm^3 (Neto, Oliveira, Correia, & Ferreira, 2008). The relatively poor spatial resolution of PET (6 mm) and fMRI (2–3 mm) as well as the sensitivity of fMRI to air/fluid interfaces and cardiac pulsations has limited the assessment of the NAcc in many investigations. Despite these challenges, many researchers have made substantial progress in investigating cocaine-induced changes (both functional and structural in nature) within this small region. Both PET and fMRI studies of cocaine-addicted individuals have reported NAcc activation during self-reported and cue-elicited cravings as well during acute cocaine intoxication (Breiter et al., 1997; Kilts, Gross, Ely, & Drexler, 2004; Kufahl et al., 2005). In fMRI studies looking at the functional activity during acute cocaine intoxication, NAcc activity was negatively correlated with reports of feeling high and positively correlated with craving (Breiter et al., 1997; Risinger et al., 2005). This suggests that activity in the NAcc may be suppressed with acute cocaine exposure and stimulated by craving.

2.2.2 Caudate Nucleus

The caudate nucleus is part of the dorsal striatum and is fairly large and functionally heterotopic. There is some suggestion that caudate volume may be larger in cocaine users compared to controls, and may be positively correlated to problems with general attention (Ersche et al., 2011; Jacobsen, Giedd, Gottschalk, Kosten, & Krystal, 2001). The ventral aspects of the caudate are believed to be involved in limbic arousal and have high connectivity to the mPFC and OFC, whereas the dorsolateral aspects of the caudate have higher connectivity with the DLPFC and are thought to be involved in cognitive processing and habit formation (Haber & Knutson, 2010). The caudate is generally thought to be involved with motivation and goal-directed behavior (Balleine, Delgado, & Hikosaka, 2007) and is active during cue-elicited craving (Garavan et al., 2000; Kilts et al., 2004). The caudate has been shown to be activated during a simulation of stress and is likewise associated with an increase in cocaine craving (Sinha et al., 2005). The caudate also has increased BOLD signal when users report feeling the euphoric "high" during acute cocaine intoxication (Breiter et al., 1997; Risinger et al., 2005).

2.2.3 Putamen

The putamen is also part of the dorsal striatum. It is generally involved in movement and learning (Balleine et al., 2007), and its volume has also been found to be larger among cocaine users (Ide et al., 2014; Jacobsen et al., 2001). The putamen has a role in cocaine craving, with increased BOLD activity during craving following cocaine administration (Breiter et al., 1997). During a PET study of cocaine cue-induced cravings, the putamen showed increased levels of dopamine receptor occupancy (Wong et al., 2006). Alterations of the activity of the putamen have also been associated with worse cognitive performance, showing decreased BOLD signal in cocaine users compared to nonusing controls in a working memory task (Moeller et al., 2010). Similarly, hypoactivation in the putamen during the Stroop test (a task of working memory) predicted shorter length of abstinence (Brewer et al., 2008).

2.2.4 Anterior Cingulate Cortex

The anterior cingulate cortex (ACC) is part of the limbic system and is involved in the regulation of attention and emotion, inhibitory control, error monitoring, and motivation (Bush, Luu, & Posner, 2000). Cocaine users have decreased gray matter density in the ACC compared to controls

(Matochik et al., 2003), and this reduction has been found to be greater for those with a longer history of abuse (Ersche et al., 2011; Franklin et al., 2002). In addition, numerous reports have demonstrated that cocaine users have lower rates of glucose usage as measured with fluorodeoxyglucose and PET, particularly in frontal regions including the cingulate gyri and OFC (Goldstein et al., 2004; Goldstein & Volkow, 2002; Volkow et al., 1991, 1992, 2005). Depressed functional activity in the ACC has been reported to persist for up to 3 (Volkow et al., 1993) to 5 months (Hanlon, Beveridge, & Porrino, 2013) of abstinence. The ACC is also associated with increased BOLD signal during craving following cocaine intoxication (Garavan et al., 2000; Maas et al., 1998; Risinger et al., 2005) and positively correlated with the "rush" of cocaine (Breiter et al., 1997; Risinger et al., 2005). Chronic cocaine users have decreased BOLD signal relative to nonusers in the ACC when completing a task requiring cognitive inhibition (Hester & Garavan, 2004; Kaufman et al., 2003) and visual attention (Kubler et al., 2005). For instance, abstinent cocaine users in treatment, compared to controls, had less ACC activation when experiencing a stressful memory indicating a lack of ability to control or inhibit the stress (Sinha et al., 2005).

2.2.5 Insula

The insula is a cortical structure located deep in the brain between the frontal and the temporal lobes. The insula has structural connections with many of the areas involved in addiction, including the amygdala, basal ganglia, thalamus, OFC, and PFC, suggesting an important role in the neural circuitry of cocaine abuse (Singer, Critchley, & Preuschoff, 2009). The insula is thought to be involved in emotion processing and arousal including awareness of one's own bodily states as well as decision-making and other executive processes. Insula volume has been found to be reduced among cocaine users, and longer use of cocaine is correlated to smaller volume of the insula (Ersche et al., 2011). In addition, smaller insula volume among cocaine users and abstainers is associated with impairments in attentional control (Ersche et al., 2011; Hanlon et al., 2011). Multiple imaging modalities (such as PET and fMRI) have also shown increased activation of the insula during acute cocaine intoxication as well as cocaine craving (Bonson et al., 2002; Kilts et al., 2001; Risinger et al., 2005).

2.2.6 Thalamus

The thalamus is one of the most highly interconnected brain regions, serving as a hub for the majority of incoming sensory information, and a relay between the striatum, pallidum, and prefrontal cortical areas. Structural studies suggest that thalamic gray matter volume is lower among chronic cocaine users than nonusing controls (Sim et al., 2007). BOLD activity in the thalamus has been associated with the euphoric state in acute cocaine intoxication (Breiter et al., 1997; Risinger et al., 2005) and during cocaine cue exposure (Garavan et al., 2000). Similarly, cocaine users have been found to have decreased BOLD signal in the thalamus during visual attention and memory tasks (Moeller et al., 2010; Tomasi et al., 2007a). Furthermore, deactivation of the thalamus during a working memory task has been associated with decreased abstinence during treatment (Moeller et al., 2010).

2.2.7 Ventral Tegmental Area

The ventral tegmental area (VTA) is a structure in the midbrain which sends dopaminergic neural projections to both the limbic and cortical areas (ie, the mesolimbic and mesocortical circuits, respectively). The VTA is a small structure and difficult to image, so activity related to this region is seldom reported in imaging studies on cocaine abuse. During a mental fatigue task, nonusing controls show enhanced activity in midbrain dopaminergic structures, including the VTA; however, this is lost in cocaine users who show a decrease in activity (Moeller, Tomasi, Honorio, Volkow, & Goldstein, 2012). Following cocaine administration in the scanner, activation in the VTA has been positively correlated with the feeling of euphoria reported by cocaine users (Breiter et al., 1997). However, VTA BOLD signal decreases during acute cocaine intoxication (Kufahl et al., 2005); this is in line with the previous work showing reductions in glucose metabolism in the VTA (London et al., 1990). In considering cue responses without delivery of the drug, one group found positive activity within the VTA, in addition to areas such as the mPFC and ACC which are commonly associated with cues (Goudriaan, Veltman, van den Brink, Dom, & Schmaal, 2013). Consistent with these findings is increased BOLD response to drug cues (Goldstein et al., 2009).

2.2.8 Amygdala

The amygdala is a subcortical structure that receives inputs from the thalamus and hippocampus and sends projections to the NAcc; it functions in the interpretation of sensory information and reinforcement (Davis & Whalen, 2001). The amygdala also directs attention and emotional responses, memory formation, and instrumental behavior. While initial studies reported that amygdala volume was smaller among cocaine users (Makris et al., 2004), this was not replicable in larger studies (Mei, Xu, Carroll, & Potenza, 2015; Xu et al., 2014). Increased amygdala activation in response to implicit cocaine cues has been correlated with positive affective response ratings to the cues, demonstrating its importance in identification of the salience of drug-related stimuli even outside of awareness (Childress et al., 2008). Despite no significant differences in volume, Mei et al. did find a negative relationship in cocaine users between amygdala volume and measures of impulsivity (Mei et al., 2015). Activation in the amygdala is increased during cue-elicited craving (Bonson et al., 2002; Childress et al., 1999; Kilts et al., 2001; Kufahl et al., 2005). Using PET, Childress and colleagues found increases in cerebral blood flow in both the amygdala and ACC in cocaine users vs controls while viewing cocaine-related video cues (Childress et al., 1999) and more recent work similarly shows increased dopamine binding within the amygdala in response to cue videos (Fotros et al., 2013). As a whole, these data support the widely held hypothesis that increased connectivity between the hippocampus, amygdala, VTA, and NAcc contributes to drug-seeking behavior (Volkow, Wang, Fowler, Tomasi, & Telang, 2011).

2.2.9 Hippocampus

The hippocampus is a midbrain structure which has long been thought to have a critical role in learning, memory, and imagination. Unlike the prefrontal cortex, the volume of the hippocampus is not typically lower in cocaine users compared to nonusers (Makris et al., 2004; Mei et al., 2015; Xu et al., 2014), although one group has found that hippocampal volume in individuals entering treatment was prospectively associated with greater drug use (Xu et al., 2014). Curiously, the hippocampus is one of the very few regions that exhibit neurogenesis in the adult human brain (Eriksson et al., 1998); blocking this neurogenesis in rodents leads to increased cocaine self-administration (Noonan, Bulin, Fuller, & Eisch, 2010). Further preclinical work has shown that the hippocampus (along with the amygdala) is involved in stress and cocaine cue-induced reinstatement (Atkins, Mashhoon, & Kantak, 2008; Belujon & Grace, 2011; Fuchs, Eaddy, Su, & Bell, 2007; Fuchs et al., 2005; Rogers & See, 2007; See, 2005). Additionally, there is greater cerebral metabolism in the right hippocampus when individuals view cocaine videos compared to neutral videos (Fotros et al., 2013).

These cross-sectional studies have demonstrated pervasive abnormalities in both cortical and subcortical structures. With this knowledge, the next pressing goal is to evaluate whether neuroimaging differences are predictive of treatment outcomes. In addition to the preliminary studies which follow, the National Institute of Health has initiated the longitudinal Adolescent Brain and Cognitive Development Study, which will follow 10,000 adolescents (all 9 or 10 years old) for 5–10 years. In addition to analysis of how drug use patterns affect typical brain development, the study will also evaluate whether there are brain-based biomarkers that are associated with vulnerability to initial use illicit drugs, escalating use patterns, and risk of relapse.

3. PREDICTING RELAPSE

Watson describing how he weaned Sherlock Holmes off of cocaine: "I was well aware that the fiend was not dead but sleeping; and I have known that the sleep was a light one and the waking near in periods of idleness."

The Adventure of the Missing Three Quarter (1904, written 1896)

In order to evaluate potential neuroimaging biomarkers, it is important to recall that addiction exists on a continuum beginning with initial drug use and progressing to habitual use, (hopefully) to abstinence and (unfortunately) often to relapse. Longitudinal assessments with fMRI typically analyze either resting state patterns or the circuit activation which occurs during tasks designed to engage certain canonical networks (ie, limbic or frontostriatal circuits) (Table 1).

3.1 Resting State Imaging Studies

Even when unengaged in activity (ie, "at rest"), activity occurs between different brain regions. The basic technique of resting state fMRI involves measurement of the spontaneous fluctuations in the BOLD signal over a period of time (Gusnard, Raichle, & Raichle, 2001), which is an indirect measure of neuronal activity. Several analytic techniques can then be used to characterize the connectivity between brain regions. Seed-based connectivity analyses compare the strength of the correlation between a preidentified region of interest and voxels in all of the other areas. Other frameworks, such as dynamic causal modeling and graph theory, are used to reveal the complex interactions of brain networks. Independent component analysis involves separating the whole brain BOLD signal timecourse into spatially distinct networks (each made up of multiple brain regions), with each network associated with a unique pattern of activity over time. In nonusing controls at rest, this has yielded a set of canonical networks with high reliability (Damoiseaux et al., 2006). Together these methods represent

Table 1 Studies That Have Investigated Neuroimaging as a Potential Biomarker for Treatment Outcome in Cocaine Users

Study	Task	User Sample	Abstainer/Relapse or Continuous Variable	Controls	Domain	When was Data Collected?	Follow-Up Time Frame
Kosten et al. (2006)	Cue and neutral videos	17	8/9	n/a	Limbic	After 2 weeks of cocaine abstinence, before any treatment	10 weeks
Brewer et al. (2008)	Stroop (color-word)	20	CV (% UDS, self-report, treatment retention)	n/a	Executive	After an average of 5.35 days abstinence	8 weeks
Moeller et al. (2010)	Delayed memory task	14	CV (TES, treatment retention)	19	Executive	Before entering treatment	16 weeks
Jia et al. (2011)	Monetary incentive delay	20	CV (UDS, self-report, treatment retention)	20	Limbic	Before first treatment session	8 weeks
Moeller et al. (2012)	Stroop (drug-word)	15	8/7	13	Limbic	After 3 week detox, and follow-up	6 months
Luo et al. (2013)	Stop signal	97	17/80	n/a	Executive	After 2–4 weeks abs in a monitoring unit	90 days
Marhe, Luijten, van de Wetering, Smits, and Franken (2013)	Stroop (drug-word)	26	CV (UDS, self-report)	n/a	Executive	4 days after entering detox treatment	3 months
Mitchell et al. (2013)	Stroop (color-word)	15	CV (UDS, self-report abs.)	15	Executive	Before beginning treatment	6/12 weeks

Continued

Table 1 Studies That Have Investigated Neuroimaging as a Potential Biomarker for Treatment Outcome in Cocaine Users—cont'd

Study	Task	User Sample	Abstainer/Relapse or Continuous Variable	Controls	Domain	When was Data Collected?	Follow-Up Time Frame
Prisciandaro et al. (2013)	Cues, go no-go task	30	24/6	N/a	Limbic	Within 1 week of entry into trial	1 week
Worhunsky et al. (2013)	Stroop (color-word)	20	CV (UDS, self-report, treatment retention)	20	Executive	After an average of 5.35 days abstinence	8 weeks
Camchong et al. (2014)	Resting state	18	12/6	15	Resting	After 5 and 13 weeks residential treatment	6 months
Clark et al. (2014)	Oddball task	45	22/23	n/a	Executive	After 1 weeks abstinence	6 months
McHugh et al. (2014)	Resting state	45	21/24	22	Resting	Final week of Treatment	30 days
Adinoff et al. (2015)	Resting state	40	22/18	21	Resting	Final week of Treatment	30 days
Contreras-Rodríguez et al. (2015)	Resting state	20	11/9	21	Resting	After 15 days abstinence	12 weeks
Balodis et al. (2016)	Monetary incentive delay	29	CV (UDS)	28	Limbic	Pre- and posttreatment	Up to 1 year

a suite of approaches that are able to measure and quantify the connectivity of brain networks.

Alterations in the resting state functional connectivity have been noted in individuals with chronic substance use (Gu et al., 2010; Kelly et al., 2011; Ma et al., 2010). For instance, connectivity between subcortical structures (eg, the VTA, hippocampus, ACC, amygdala, and thalamus) was decreased during resting state fMRI in cocaine users. Furthermore, weakened connectivity strength between the VTA, the thalamus, and NAcc was correlated with more years of cocaine use (Gu et al., 2010). Other groups have found reductions in interhemispheric connectivity, with differences that localize to frontal regions associated with executive control, motor planning, and response inhibition (Kelly et al., 2011). These findings are consistent with theories which suggest that addiction pathology is related to deficits in various components of neurocognition.

The functional connectivity between the NAcc and the subgenual ACC (sgACC) has been shown to correlate with successful abstinence. One study of cocaine users used seed-based analysis of fMRI scans taken after 5 and 13 weeks of abstinence in a residential treatment center; at the 5-week mark, higher functional connectivity between the NAcc, the left PFC, and PCC was associated with higher rates of relapse, as was higher functional connectivity between the PFC and the sgACC (Camchong et al., 2014). These results should be interpreted with caution as another study of 45 individuals placed seeds in similar regions but failed to find significant connectivity differences between the 24 individuals that relapsed and the 21 that remained abstinent (McHugh et al., 2013). Additionally, there are indications that stronger connectivity between the basolateral amygdala and the precuneus, lingual and parahippocampal gyrus, along with weaker connectivity between the corticomedial amygdala and the vmPFC is a powerful predictor of relapse (McHugh et al., 2014). Increased functional connectivity between the hippocampus, the posterior cingulate gyrus, and the precuneus was shown in a pseudocontinuous arterial spin labeling study (a technique similar to fMRI in which regional blood flow is interpreted as an indirect marker of synaptic activity) to be associated with relapse, with 75% accuracy (Adinoff et al., 2015); these findings were also reproducible using single-photon emission computed tomography technology (Adinoff, Harris, Gu, & Stein, 2016). This proposed hippocampal hyperactivity supports previous structural imaging studies in which hippocampal volume was positively associated with a return to drug use (Xu et al., 2014). Overall, when neural networks are examined at rest (ie, intrinsic network connectivity), greater connectivity within typical limbic- and reward-related circuitry is associated with worse outcomes, suggesting that the network tone is too high.

3.2 Neuroimaging During Limbic System Activating Tasks

Previous cross-sectional analyses have identified drug-induced limbic circuit abnormalities in addiction (Volkow et al., 1991, 1992, 2005). These alterations can be investigated through the use of neuroimaging while exposing cocaine users to images or videos that are hypothetically associated with drug use (ie, images of drugs or other paraphernalia). In nonusers, these images will reliably activate visual areas of the brain, but in cocaine users (present or former), there is increased activation in several brain regions, particularly in areas associated with reward (Wilcox, Teshiba, Merideth, Ling, & Mayer, 2011). Activity in the left precentral gyrus, posterior cingulate, the right lingual gyrus, inferior occipital gyrus, and the superior temporal gyrus correlated with the increased abstinence (Kosten et al., 2006); furthermore, increased activity in the posterior cingulate cortex significantly differentiated those that relapsed from those that did not.

The monetary incentive delay task has been combined with fMRI to explore circuit activation during simulations of reward and punishment; brain activation can be analyzed during the reward prediction, anticipation, and outcome processing portions associated with the task (Knutson, Westdorp, Kaiser, & Hommer, 2000). When cocaine users were tested at baseline, increased activity between the bilateral thalamus and right putamen was associated with decreased ability to maintain abstinence after 8 weeks of substance abuse treatment (Jia et al., 2011). Additionally, activation of the left amygdala and parahippocampal gyrus was associated with increased rates of treatment dropout (Jia et al., 2011); similarly the right thalamus, ventral striatum, and left putamen were inversely correlated with abstinence. Elevated activity in the NAcc in response to simulation of monetary loss was associated with decreased abstinence (Balodis et al., 2016). In agreement with the resting state data, these studies add to the evidence that elevated activity and connectivity with the limbic reward system (particularly the NAcc) are associated with poor outcomes in treatment (Fig. 2).

3.3 Neuroimaging During Executive System Activating Tasks

Drug use has been associated with deficits in neurocognition, such as poor working memory (Tomasi et al., 2007b), difficulty in attentional shifting (Kubler et al., 2005), and response inhibition and mental flexibility

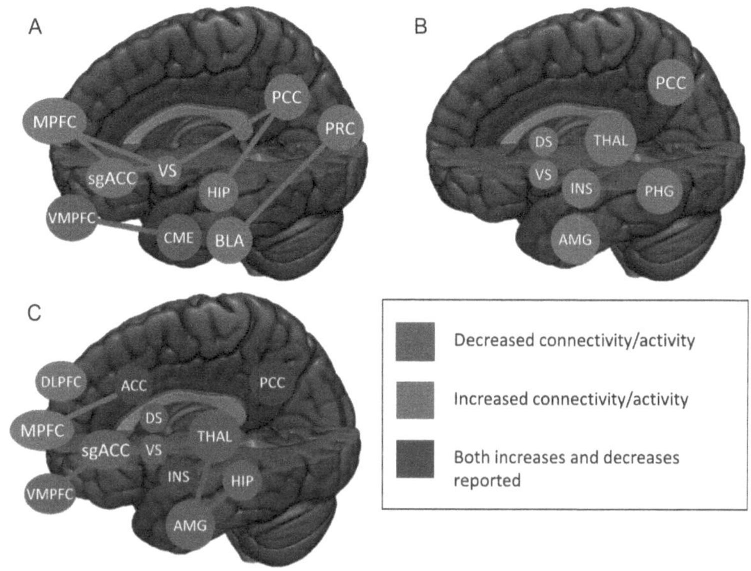

Fig. 2 Regional brain connectivity or activity that was associated with poor treatment outcomes. (A) Results from seed-based connectivity during resting state. (B) Activation related to poor outcomes during limbic-associated tasks is consistently elevated. (C) Reduced activation during tasks measuring executive function was associated with worse outcomes, though cortical regions associated with internal state and self-reflection show mixed responses. *ACC*, anterior cingulate Cortex; *AMG*, amygdala; *BLA*, basolateral amygdala; *CME*, corticomedial amygdala; *DS*, dorsal striatum; *HIP*, hippocampus; *INS*, insula; *MPFC*, medial prefrontal cortex; *PCC*, posterior cingulate cortex; *PHG*, parahippocampal gyrus; *PRC*, precuneus; *sgACC*, subgenual anterior cingulate cortex; *THAL*, thalamus; *vmPFC*, ventromedial prefrontal cortex; *VS*, ventral striatum.

(Verdejo-García, Bechara, Recknor, & Pérez-García, 2006). However, these tests of neurocognition have not been well validated as predictors of treatment success; consequently, the addition of brain imaging is being explored as a means of improving outcome predictability.

3.3.1 Attention

Initial neurocognitive testing using the Stroop task previously revealed that attentional deficits are correlated with increased treatment dropout (Streeter et al., 2008). However, a similar study using a modified version of the Stroop task (which contained drug cue words) failed to find a relationship between ability to maintain attention and cocaine relapse (Kennedy, Gross, Ely, Drexler, & Kilts, 2014). To further explore the relationship between attentional capability and treatment engagement, Brewer and colleagues (2008) found that individuals with longer reaction times in the Stroop task remained enrolled in treatment significantly longer, though there was no relationship between behavioral performance and abstinence as measured by urine drug screens (Brewer et al., 2008).

From a neuroimaging perspective, Brewer et al. (2008) also demonstrated that decreased activity in the right putamen during the Stroop task was associated with increased cocaine use. Exploratory analysis revealed a negative correlation between activity in the left DLPFC and weeks in treatment, such that the less activated this region was, the better the outcomes (Brewer et al., 2008). Independent component analysis was applied to this same data set to derive networks activated during the task, including the cingulo-opercular, fronto-parietal, fronto-cingular, subcortical, and fronto-striatal networks (Worhunsky et al., 2013). Of these five networks, only three were correlated with treatment outcomes: increased activation of the fronto-cingular network (which included the ACC, the medial and middle frontal regions, and the dorsal insula) was associated with decreased treatment retention; decreased recruitment of the subcortical network (which consisted of the thalamus, striatum, amygdala, hippocampus, and left inferior frontal cortex) was associated with decreased abstinence; and deactivation of the ventral fronto-striatal network (which included the vmPFC, subgenual, and rostral ACC) was associated with increased drug use during treatment. An intrinsic connectivity distribution analysis involving the Stroop task (an imaging analysis technique similar to independent component analysis) found decreased connectivity in the thalamus, ventral striatum, substantia nigra, right insula, and left hippocampus was associated with lower levels of abstinence (Mitchell et al., 2013). Together these data suggest that poor outcomes in cocaine treatment programs are associated with dopaminergic and limbic dysfunction, even when investigating neural engagement in an executive control task.

3.3.2 Response Inhibition

The ability to control an impulsive response is another aspect of cognition that is believed to be abnormal in drug use; the oddball, stop-signal, and go/no-go tasks are three assessment tools commonly used to measure this cognitive function during tests of attention. In a study utilizing the oddball task (in which individuals are exposed to a stream of repetitive stimuli that is intermittently punctuated by novel stimuli), the BOLD response to distracting stimuli was significantly higher in the posterior cingulate cortex, right insula, and ACC and reliably dissociated the relapsing group from the abstinent group (Clark et al., 2014); these findings were overall consistent with similar previous work using the oddball task (Bauer, 1997). Similar studies using the go/no-go task found that a difference in activity within the precentral gyrus differentiated those who used cocaine prior to a 1-week follow-up (Prisciandaro, Myrick, Henderson, McRae-Clark, & Brady, 2013). In a study of working memory, thalamic deactivation was associated with worse treatment outcomes (Moeller et al., 2010). Repeated reports of the involvement of the PCC in multiple studies are of interest, given its functional relationships with the DLPFC, other regions of the cognitive network (Yu et al., 2011), and limbic areas, including the subgenual cingulate cortex (Vogt, Vogt, & Laureys, 2006) and insula (Cauda et al., 2011). Overall, these data suggest that neurocognitive deficits in executive function and increased limbic-related responses are associated with increased rates of relapse.

3.4 Moving Forward

In the future, studies should consider the potential bias that occurs by selection of seed regions (such as the striatum, amygdala, and hippocampus); the use of ICA to analyze resting state data might reveal more significant contributions of frontal brain regions. Beyond new analyses on existing data sets, there is a need to test predictors on independent data. Resting state fMRI shows great promise, as the lack of task constraints makes these existing data sets ideal for comparing between laboratories. A larger challenge faced by the field is the attempt to describe and standardize treatment strategies and treatment outcomes. Consensus on the best dependent measures to use, crucial time points to examine subjects during treatment, and the types of comorbidities acceptable for enrollment would improve analysis and interpretation of neuroimaging data. This information would further pave the road toward development of more effective treatment modalities which attenuate or activate activity in key regions.

4. FROM BRAIN TO BEDSIDE—DEVELOPING NEURAL CIRCUIT-BASED TREATMENTS FOR SUBSTANCE DEPENDENCE

The theories which I have expressed there, and which appear to you to be so chimerical, are really extremely practical—so practical that I depend upon them for my bread and cheese.

A Study in Scarlet, Sherlock Holmes (Doyle, 1887)

There is no FDA-approved *pharmacotherapy* for treating cocaine use disorder. There is also no consistent standard of care in terms of treating cocaine-dependent individuals with *behavioral therapy*. Behavioral interventions commonly used by psychiatrists and clinical psychologist include contingency management (in which patients are rewarded for maintaining sobriety) and cognitive behavioral therapy (in which patients learn to control and adjust behaviors that lead to drug taking). Although behavioral therapies can play an important role in supporting abstinence, studies indicate that their efficacy is low to moderate depending on the substance of abuse (Dutra et al., 2008).

Recent animal studies using molecular and optogenetic techniques suggest that modifying activity of fronto-striatal circuits (perhaps through the use of brain stimulation techniques) can attenuate, if not completely abolish, cocaine seeking. With accumulating knowledge about disrupted functional connectivity in limbic and executive control circuits in cocaine users, the clinical neuroscience community is now in the process of developing non-invasive brain stimulation treatments designed to restore healthy function in these circuits, one of which is transcranial magnetic stimulation (TMS).

4.1 Transcranial Magnetic Stimulation

An FDA-approved treatment for major depressive disorder since 2008, TMS, is currently being evaluated as a treatment for craving for a number of substance use disorders. This technique is a noninvasive form of brain stimulation which induces a depolarization of neurons through electromagnetic induction. The potential of TMS as a new tool for modulating craving among substance-dependent populations has garnered significant attention from both the National Institute of Health (NIH) and in the literature (see reviews: Barr et al., 2011; Bellamoli et al., 2014; Feil & Zangen, 2010; Gorelick, Zangen, & George, 2014; Wing et al., 2013). When integrated with MRI, a single pulse of TMS induces an elevation in the BOLD signal in the area under the coil and in monosynaptic target regions (Bohning et al., 1998). The amplitude of the BOLD signal induced by a single pulse of TMS to the primary motor cortex is not significantly different than the amplitude of the BOLD signal induced by an individual instructed to squeeze his/her hand in a manner that mimics the TMS evoked muscle contraction (Denslow, Lomarev, George, & Bohning, 2005). This correspondence between the TMS-evoked (external) BOLD signal and the voluntarily evoked (internal) BOLD signal produced by a participant is important when considering how a TMS-evoked BOLD signal in the prefrontal cortex may mimic the BOLD signal evoked by an internal craving state or external cue exposure. Through the use of MRI during TMS, we recently demonstrated that it is possible to differentially activate fronto-striatal circuits involved in limbic control from those involved in executive control through stimulating the MPFC and DLPFC, respectively (Hanlon et al., 2013).

TMS can also be used to induce either long-term depression (LTD) or long-term potentiation (LTP) of specific circuits by applying different stimulation parameters to distinct cortical brain regions (reviewed in Fitzgerald, Fountain, & Daskalakis, 2006; Thickbroom, 2007). An LTD-like effect can be achieved using TMS by using either low-frequency stimulation (typically 1 Hz) or continuous theta burst (Huang, Edwards, Rounis, Bhatia, & Rothwell, 2005). While the LTP component of stimulation remains unclear, Stagg and colleagues have demonstrated through imaging methods that the attenuating effect of cTBS is likely due to an increase in γ-aminobutyric acid at the area of stimulation (Stagg et al., 2009).

4.2 Potential Neural Targets for Addiction

As previously discussed, high rates of relapse in cocaine users may be due to dysfunction of the executive control loop as well as the limbic circuitry. In a nonaddicted state, the executive control loop acts to resist the limbic circuitry-related craving for the drug. However with chronic cocaine use, there is elevation in the cue-related functional activity within limbic neural circuitry (Ersche et al., 2011; Moeller et al., 2001) and depressed activity in the executive control loop (Goldstein et al., 2004; Kubler et al., 2005; Moeller et al., 2010). Thus, selective modulation of fronto-striatal circuits to treat addiction requires either increasing the strength of the executive control network or decreasing the engagement of limbic reward circuit when an individual is presented with cocaine cues (Fig. 3).

4.2.1 Increase in Executive Control Network Activity

To date, nearly all rTMS studies in addiction have targeted the same neural region: the DLPFC (Camprodon, Martinez-Raga, Alonso-Alonso, Shih, & Pascual-Leone, 2007; Eichhammer et al., 2003; Herremans et al., 2012; Hoppner, Broese, Wendler, Berger, & Thome, 2011; Li et al., 2013; Mishra, Nizamie, Das, & Praharaj, 2010; Politi, Fauci, Santoro, & Smeraldi, 2008; Pripfl, Tomova, Riecansky, & Lamm, 2014). While many of these studies demonstrated that high-frequency (LTP-like) rTMS

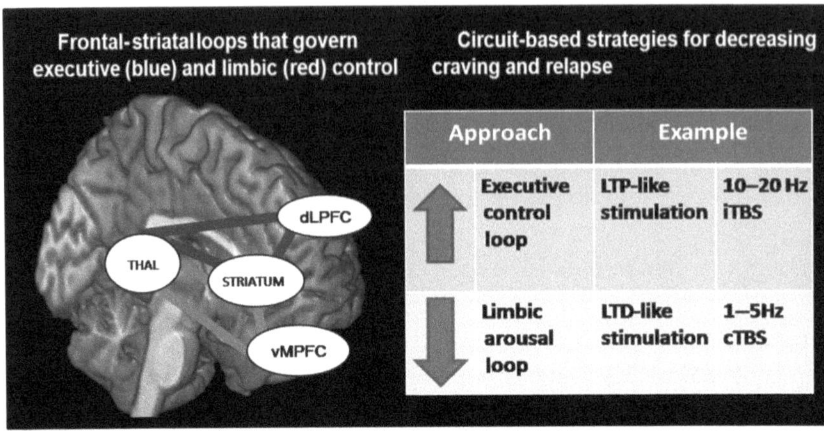

Fig. 3 Potential strategies for developing novel brain stimulation treatment strategies for addiction which leverage our knowledge of neural circuit irregularities that contribute to relapse among treatment-seeking cocaine users.

stimulation to the DLPFC can result in a significant reduction of craving, the neurobiological mechanism through which this might happen is not clear. In a comprehensive review of the literature on the efficacy of rTMS as a treatment tool for smoking, Wing and colleagues presented a model in which the beneficial effects of LTP-like TMS on the DLPFC are associated with a release of dopamine in the NAcc (Wing et al., 2013). This model is supported by the work of Strafella and colleagues which used PET to demonstrate that DLPFC stimulation was associated with an increase in dopamine binding in the caudate (Strafella, Paus, Barrett, & Dagher, 2001).

4.2.2 Decrease in Reward Network Activity

The primary cortical input to the NAcc however is not the DLPFC, but rather, the mPFC and OFC. Given that the NAcc is one of the primary brain regions involved in craving, targeting the mPFC would be a more direct method to modulate NAcc activity in substance-dependent populations. Further, given that craving for cocaine is associated with an increase in dopamine in the striatum, it is reasonable to pursue an LTD-like rTMS protocol over the mPFC to attenuate activity in this neural circuit. Prior data from our laboratory demonstrates that a single TMS pulse of the mPFC in non-using individuals lead to an increase in BOLD signal in the ventral striatum (Hanlon, Canterberry, et al., 2013).

Furthermore, continuous theta burst TMS stimulation of the vmPFC can decrease BOLD signal in both the vmPFC and the NAcc of chronic

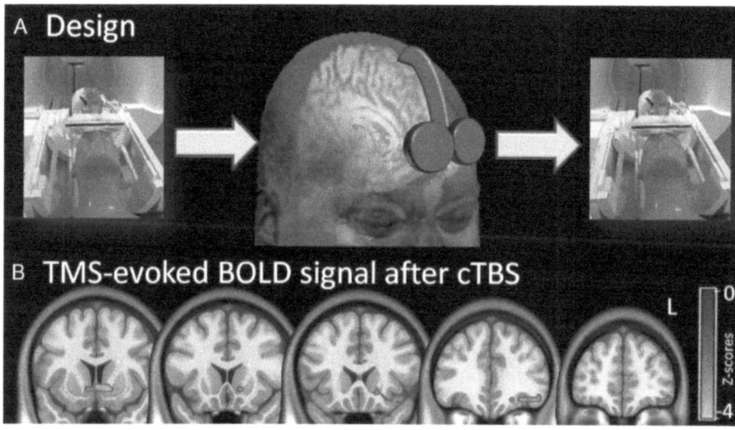

Fig. 4 The effects of continuous theta burst stimulation (*cTBS*) to the *left* vmPFC/OFC in cocaine users. Interleaved TMS/BOLD imaging was used to measure TMS-evoked BOLD signal immediately before and after cocaine users were given a dose of cTBS to the *left* frontal pole (A). The TMS coil was placed over FP1 (EEG: 10–20 system) for both the interleaved TMS/BOLD scan (*left* and *right panel*) and the cTBS session (*center panel*). The *red* (*gray* in the print version) area represents the region of interest to which the coil is targeted (AAL: left superior and middle orbital prefrontal cortex inferior to the anterior commissure). Real cTBS (LTD-like) led to a significant decrease in BOLD signal in the *left* orbital/medial prefrontal cortex and ventral striatum (SPM8, $p < 0.05$ family-wise error correction, negative *Z*-scores shown). (B) The cTBS protocol was two trains of 1800 pulses, 110% RMT, 60 s intertrain interval, intensity ramped from 80% to 110% over first 30 s. *L*, left hemisphere. *Adapted from Hanlon, C. A., Dowdle, L. T., Austelle, C. W., DeVries, W., Mithoefer, O., Badran, B. W., & George, M. S. (2015). What goes up, can come down: Novel brain stimulation paradigms may attenuate craving and craving-related neural circuitry in substance dependent individuals.* Brain Research, 1628*(Pt. A), 199–209. doi: 10.1016/j.brainres.2015.02.053.*

cocaine users (Hanlon et al., 2015) (Fig. 4). In a follow-up study which examined the effects of continuous theta burst stimulation on cocaine cue-evoked brain activity, one notable finding was that there was significant individual variability in TMS treatment response; this was related to baseline variance in striatal network engagement when participants viewed cocaine-related visual cues. Specifically, individuals that had higher striatal activity when viewing cocaine cues demonstrated a more pronounced attenuation of striatal activity to cues following the cTBS sessions. Conversely, individuals with low striatal engagement during cocaine cues had an elevated response following continuous TBS. These data highlight the importance of considering individual variability in future clinical trials of TMS as a treatment adjuvant to behavioral therapy for cocaine dependence. Another research goal is to determine if a positive treatment response can be prospectively predicted. Additionally, before studying this paradigm in large (and expensive) clinical trials, it is critical to determine whether this treatment is even well tolerated, feasible, and associated with improved outcomes such as abstinence and decreased cravings.

4.3 Future Directions

While these studies are by no means exhaustive, they convey an attempt to identify neuroimaging biomarkers that can be used to predict successful abstinence from cocaine. What they do not convey is the wealth of potential that neuroimaging also portends such as personalized treatment programs and preventive screening for predisposition to addiction. It is clear, however, that neuroimaging has an important role play as the field of addiction medicine moves to bridge neurobiological findings from preclinical studies to effective treatment strategies.

REFERENCES

Adinoff, B., Gu, H., Merrick, C., McHugh, M., Jeon-Slaughter, H., Lu, H., ... Stein, E. A. (2015). Basal hippocampal activity and its functional connectivity predicts cocaine relapse. *Biological Psychiatry, 78*(7), 496–504. http://dx.doi.org/10.1016/j.biopsych.2014.12.027.

Adinoff B., Harris T.S., Gu H., & Stein E.A. (2016). Posterior hippocampal regional cerebral blood flow predicts abstinence: A replication study, *Addiction Biology*, in press, http://dx.doi.org/10.1111/adb.12361.

Afonso, L., Mohammad, T., & Thatai, D. (2007). Crack whips the heart: A review of the cardiovascular toxicity of cocaine. *American Journal of Cardiology, 100*(6), 1040–1043. http://dx.doi.org/10.1016/j.amjcard.2007.04.049.

Atkins, A. L., Mashhoon, Y., & Kantak, K. M. (2008). Hippocampal regulation of contextual cue-induced reinstatement of cocaine-seeking behavior. *Pharmacology Biochemistry and Behavior, 90*(3), 481–491. http://dx.doi.org/10.1016/j.pbb.2008.04.007.

Balleine, B. W., Delgado, M. R., & Hikosaka, O. (2007). The role of the dorsal striatum in reward and decision-making. *Journal of Neuroscience, 27*(31), 8161–8165. http://dx.doi.org/10.1523/JNEUROSCI.1554-07.2007.

Balodis, I. M., Kober, H., Worhunsky, P. D., Stevens, M. C., Pearlson, G. D., Carroll, K. M., & Potenza, M. N. (2016). Neurofunctional reward processing changes in cocaine dependence during recovery. *Neuropsychopharmacology, 41*, 2112–2121. http://dx.doi.org/10.1038/npp.2016.11.

Barr, M. S., Farzan, F., Wing, V. C., George, T. P., Fitzgerald, P. B., & Daskalakis, Z. J. (2011). Repetitive transcranial magnetic stimulation and drug addiction. *International Review of Psychiatry, 23*(5), 454–466. http://dx.doi.org/10.3109/09540261.2011.618827.

Bauer, L. O. (1997). Frontal P300 decrements, childhood conduct disorder, family history, and the prediction of relapse among abstinent cocaine abusers. *Drug and Alcohol Dependence, 44*(1), 1–10.

Bellamoli, E., Manganotti, P., Schwartz, R. P., Rimondo, C., Gomma, M., & Serpelloni, G. (2014). rTMS in the treatment of drug addiction: An update about human studies. *Behavioural Neurology, 2014*, 815215. http://dx.doi.org/10.1155/2014/815215.

Belujon, P., & Grace, A. A. (2011). Hippocampus, amygdala, and stress: Interacting systems that affect susceptibility to addiction. *Annals of the New York Academy of Sciences*, *1216*, 114–121. http://dx.doi.org/10.1111/j.1749-6632.2010.05896.x.

Boghdadi, M. S., & Henning, R. J. (1997). Cocaine: Pathophysiology and clinical toxicology. *Heart & Lung*, *26*(6), 466–483. http://dx.doi.org/10.1016/S0147-9563(97)90040-6. quiz 484–465.

Bohning, D. E., Shastri, A., Nahas, Z., Lorberbaum, J. P., Andersen, S. W., Dannels, W. R., ... George, M. S. (1998). Echoplanar BOLD fMRI of brain activation induced by concurrent transcranial magnetic stimulation. *Investigative Radiology*, *33*(6), 336–340.

Bolla, K. I., Eldreth, D. A., London, E. D., Kiehl, K. A., Mouratidis, M., Contoreggi, C., ... Ernst, M. (2003). Orbitofrontal cortex dysfunction in abstinent cocaine abusers performing a decision-making task. *Neuroimage*, *19*(3), 1085–1094.

Bonson, K. R., Grant, S. J., Contoreggi, C. S., Links, J. M., Metcalfe, J., Weyl, H. L., ... London, E. D. (2002). Neural systems and cue-induced cocaine craving. *Neuropsychopharmacology*, *26*(3), 376–386. http://dx.doi.org/10.1016/S0893-133X(01)00371-2.

Breiter, H. C., Gollub, R. L., Weisskoff, R. M., Kennedy, D. N., Makris, N., Berke, J. D., ... Hyman, S. E. (1997). Acute effects of cocaine on human brain activity and emotion. *Neuron*, *19*(3), 591–611.

Brewer, J. A., Worhunsky, P. D., Carroll, K. M., Rounsaville, B. J., & Potenza, M. N. (2008). Pretreatment brain activation during stroop task is associated with outcomes in cocaine-dependent patients. *Biological Psychiatry*, *64*(11), 998–1004. http://dx.doi.org/10.1016/j.biopsych.2008.05.024.

Bush, G., Luu, P., & Posner, M. I. (2000). Cognitive and emotional influences in anterior cingulate cortex. *Trends in Cognitive Science*, *4*(6), 215–222.

Camchong, J., Macdonald, A. W., 3rd, Mueller, B. A., Nelson, B., Specker, S., Slaymaker, V., & Lim, K. O. (2014). Changes in resting functional connectivity during abstinence in stimulant use disorder: A preliminary comparison of relapsers and abstainers. *Drug and Alcohol Dependence*, *139*, 145–151. http://dx.doi.org/10.1016/j.drugalcdep.2014.03.024.

Camprodon, J. A., Martinez-Raga, J., Alonso-Alonso, M., Shih, M. C., & Pascual-Leone, A. (2007). One session of high frequency repetitive transcranial magnetic stimulation (rTMS) to the right prefrontal cortex transiently reduces cocaine craving. *Drug and Alcohol Dependence*, *86*(1), 91–94. http://dx.doi.org/10.1016/j.drugalcdep.2006.06.002.

Cauda, F., D'Agata, F., Sacco, K., Duca, S., Geminiani, G., & Vercelli, A. (2011). Functional connectivity of the insula in the resting brain. *Neuroimage*, *55*(1), 8–23. http://dx.doi.org/10.1016/j.neuroimage.2010.11.049.

Childress, A. R., Ehrman, R. N., Wang, Z., Li, Y., Sciortino, N., Hakun, J., ... O'Brien, C. P. (2008). Prelude to passion: Limbic activation by "unseen" drug and sexual cues. *PLoS One*, *3*(1), e1506. http://dx.doi.org/10.1371/journal.pone.0001506.

Childress, A. R., Mozley, P. D., McElgin, W., Fitzgerald, J., Reivich, M., & O'Brien, C. P. (1999). Limbic activation during cue-induced cocaine craving. *The American Journal of Psychiatry*, *156*(1), 11–18.

Clark, V. P., Beatty, G. K., Anderson, R. E., Kodituwakku, P., Phillips, J. P., Lane, T. D., ... Calhoun, V. D. (2014). Reduced fMRI activity predicts relapse in patients recovering from stimulant dependence. *Human Brain Mapping*, *35*(2), 414–428.

Connolly, C. G., Bell, R. P., Foxe, J. J., & Garavan, H. (2013). Dissociated grey matter changes with prolonged addiction and extended abstinence in cocaine users. *PLoS One*, *8*(3), e59645. http://dx.doi.org/10.1371/journal.pone.0059645.

Contreras-Rodríguez, O., Albein-Urios, N., Perales, J. C., Martínez-Gonzalez, J. M., Vilar-López, R., Fernández-Serrano, M. J., ... Verdejo-García, A. (2015). Cocaine-specific neuroplasticity in the ventral striatum network is linked to delay discounting and drug relapse. *Addiction*, *110*(12), 1953–1962.

Damoiseaux, J. S., Rombouts, S. A. R. B., Barkhof, F., Scheltens, P., Stam, C. J., Smith, S. M., & Beckmann, C. F. (2006). Consistent resting-state networks across healthy subjects. *Proceedings of the National Academy of Sciences of the United States of America, 103*, 13848–13853. http://dx.doi.org/10.1073/pnas.0601417103.

Davis, M., & Whalen, P. J. (2001). The amygdala: Vigilance and emotion. *Molecular Psychiatry, 6*(1), 13–34.

Denslow, S., Lomarev, M., George, M. S., & Bohning, D. E. (2005). Cortical and subcortical brain effects of transcranial magnetic stimulation (TMS)-induced movement: An interleaved TMS/functional magnetic resonance imaging study. *Biological Psychiatry, 57*(7), 752–760. http://dx.doi.org/10.1016/j.biopsych.2004.12.017.

Doyle, A. C. (1887). *A study in scarlet*. Ward & Lock Co.

Doyle, A. C. (1890). *The sign of four*. Lippincott Monthly Magazine.

Dutra, L., Stathopoulou, G., Basden, S. L., Leyro, T. M., Powers, M. B., & Otto, M. W. (2008). A meta-analytic review of psychosocial interventions for substance use disorders. *The American Journal of Psychiatry, 165*(2), 179–187. http://dx.doi.org/10.1176/appi.ajp.2007.06111851.

Eichhammer, P., Johann, M., Kharraz, A., Binder, H., Pittrow, D., Wodarz, N., & Hajak, G. (2003). High-frequency repetitive transcranial magnetic stimulation decreases cigarette smoking. *Journal of Clinical Psychiatry, 64*(8), 951–953.

Eriksson, P. S., Perfilieva, E., Bjork-Eriksson, T., Alborn, A. M., Nordborg, C., Peterson, D. A., & Gage, F. H. (1998). Neurogenesis in the adult human hippocampus. *Nature Medicine, 4*(11), 1313–1317. http://dx.doi.org/10.1038/3305.

Ersche, K. D., Barnes, A., Jones, P. S., Morein-Zamir, S., Robbins, T. W., & Bullmore, E. T. (2011). Abnormal structure of frontostriatal brain systems is associated with aspects of impulsivity and compulsivity in cocaine dependence. *Brain, 134*(Pt. 7), 2013–2024. http://dx.doi.org/10.1093/brain/awr138.

Everitt, B. J., & Robbins, T. W. (2005). Neural systems of reinforcement for drug addiction: From actions to habits to compulsion. *Nature Neuroscience, 8*(11), 1481–1489. http://dx.doi.org/10.1038/nn1579.

Feil, J., & Zangen, A. (2010). Brain stimulation in the study and treatment of addiction. *Neuroscience & Biobehavioral Reviews, 34*(4), 559–574. http://dx.doi.org/10.1016/j.neubiorev.2009.11.006.

Fein, G., Di Sclafani, V., & Meyerhoff, D. J. (2002). Prefrontal cortical volume reduction associated with frontal cortex function deficit in 6-week abstinent crack-cocaine dependent men. *Drug and Alcohol Dependence, 68*(1), 87–93.

Fitzgerald, P. B., Fountain, S., & Daskalakis, Z. J. (2006). A comprehensive review of the effects of rTMS on motor cortical excitability and inhibition. *Clinical Neurophysiology, 117*(12), 2584–2596. http://dx.doi.org/10.1016/j.clinph.2006.06.712.

Fotros, A., Casey, K. F., Larcher, K., Verhaeghe, J. A., Cox, S. M., Gravel, P., … Leyton, M. (2013). Cocaine cue-induced dopamine release in amygdala and hippocampus: A high-resolution PET [(1)(8)F]fallypride study in cocaine dependent participants. *Neuropsychopharmacology, 38*(9), 1780–1788. http://dx.doi.org/10.1038/npp.2013.77.

Franklin, T. R., Acton, P. D., Maldjian, J. A., Gray, J. D., Croft, J. R., Dackis, C. A., … Childress, A. R. (2002). Decreased gray matter concentration in the insular, orbitofrontal, cingulate, and temporal cortices of cocaine patients. *Biological Psychiatry, 51*(2), 134–142.

Fuchs, R. A., Eaddy, J. L., Su, Z. I., & Bell, G. H. (2007). Interactions of the basolateral amygdala with the dorsal hippocampus and dorsomedial prefrontal cortex regulate drug context-induced reinstatement of cocaine-seeking in rats. *European Journal of Neuroscience, 26*(2), 487–498. http://dx.doi.org/10.1111/j.1460-9568.2007.05674.x.

Fuchs, R. A., Evans, K. A., Ledford, C. C., Parker, M. P., Case, J. M., Mehta, R. H., & See, R. E. (2005). The role of the dorsomedial prefrontal cortex, basolateral amygdala, and dorsal hippocampus in contextual reinstatement of cocaine seeking in rats. *Neuropsychopharmacology*, *30*(2), 296–309. http://dx.doi.org/10.1038/sj.npp.1300579.

Garavan, H., Pankiewicz, J., Bloom, A., Cho, J. K., Sperry, L., Ross, T. J., … Stein, E. A. (2000). Cue-induced cocaine craving: Neuroanatomical specificity for drug users and drug stimuli. *The American Journal of Psychiatry*, *157*(11), 1789–1798.

Goldstein, R. Z., Leskovjan, A. C., Hoff, A. L., Hitzemann, R., Bashan, F., Khalsa, S. S., … Volkow, N. D. (2004). Severity of neuropsychological impairment in cocaine and alcohol addiction: Association with metabolism in the prefrontal cortex. *Neuropsychologia*, *42*(11), 1447–1458. http://dx.doi.org/10.1016/j.neuropsychologia.2004.04.002.

Goldstein, R. Z., Tomasi, D., Alia-Klein, N., Honorio Carrillo, J., Maloney, T., Woicik, P. A., … Volkow, N. D. (2009). Dopaminergic response to drug words in cocaine addiction. *Journal of Neuroscience*, *29*(18), 6001–6006. http://dx.doi.org/10.1523/JNEUROSCI.4247-08.2009.

Goldstein, R. Z., & Volkow, N. D. (2002). Drug addiction and its underlying neurobiological basis: Neuroimaging evidence for the involvement of the frontal cortex. *The American Journal of Psychiatry*, *159*(10), 1642–1652. http://dx.doi.org/10.1176/appi.ajp.159.10.1642.

Gorelick, D. A., Zangen, A., & George, M. S. (2014). Transcranial magnetic stimulation in the treatment of substance addiction. *Annals of the New York Academy of Sciences*, *1327*, 79–93. http://dx.doi.org/10.1111/nyas.12479.

Goudriaan, A. E., Veltman, D. J., van den Brink, W., Dom, G., & Schmaal, L. (2013). Neurophysiological effects of modafinil on cue-exposure in cocaine dependence: A randomized placebo-controlled cross-over study using pharmacological fMRI. *Addictive Behaviors*, *38*(2), 1509–1517. http://dx.doi.org/10.1016/j.addbeh.2012.04.006.

Grant, S., London, E. D., Newlin, D. B., Villemagne, V. L., Liu, X., Contoreggi, C., … Margolin, A. (1996). Activation of memory circuits during cue-elicited cocaine craving. *Proceedings of the National Academy of Sciences of the United States of America*, *93*(21), 12040–12045.

Gu, H., Salmeron, B. J., Ross, T. J., Geng, X., Zhan, W., Stein, E. A., & Yang, Y. (2010). Mesocorticolimbic circuits are impaired in chronic cocaine users as demonstrated by resting-state functional connectivity. *Neuroimage*, *53*(2), 593–601. http://dx.doi.org/10.1016/j.neuroimage.2010.06.066.

Gusnard, D. A., Raichle, M. E., & Raichle, M. E. (2001). Searching for a baseline: Functional imaging and the resting human brain. *Nature Reviews. Neuroscience*, *2*(10), 685–694. http://dx.doi.org/10.1038/35094500.

Haber, S. N., & Knutson, B. (2010). The reward circuit: Linking primate anatomy and human imaging. *Neuropsychopharmacology*, *35*(1), 4–26. http://dx.doi.org/10.1038/npp.2009.129.

Hanlon, C. A., Beveridge, T. J., & Porrino, L. J. (2013). Recovering from cocaine: Insights from clinical and preclinical investigations. *Neuroscience & Biobehavioral Reviews*, *37*(9 Pt. A), 2037–2046. http://dx.doi.org/10.1016/j.neubiorev.2013.04.007.

Hanlon, C. A., Canterberry, M., Taylor, J. J., DeVries, W., Li, X., Brown, T. R., & George, M. S. (2013). Probing the frontostriatal loops involved in executive and limbic processing via interleaved TMS and functional MRI at two prefrontal locations: A pilot study. *PLoS One*, *8*(7), e67917. http://dx.doi.org/10.1371/journal.pone.0067917.

Hanlon, C. A., Dowdle, L. T., Austelle, C. W., DeVries, W., Mithoefer, O., Badran, B. W., & George, M. S. (2015). What goes up, can come down: Novel brain stimulation paradigms may attenuate craving and craving-related neural circuitry in substance dependent individuals. *Brain Research*, *1628*(Pt. A), 199–209. http://dx.doi.org/10.1016/j.brainres.2015.02.053.

Hanlon, C. A., Dufault, D. L., Wesley, M. J., & Porrino, L. J. (2011). Elevated gray and white matter densities in cocaine abstainers compared to current users. *Psychopharmacology*, *218*(4), 681–692. http://dx.doi.org/10.1007/s00213-011-2360-y.

Herremans, S. C., Baeken, C., Vanderbruggen, N., Vanderhasselt, M. A., Zeeuws, D., Santermans, L., & De Raedt, R. (2012). No influence of one right-sided prefrontal HF-rTMS session on alcohol craving in recently detoxified alcohol-dependent patients: Results of a naturalistic study. *Drug and Alcohol Dependence, 120*(1–3), 209–213. http://dx.doi.org/10.1016/j.drugalcdep.2011.07.021.

Hester, R., & Garavan, H. (2004). Executive dysfunction in cocaine addiction: Evidence for discordant frontal, cingulate, and cerebellar activity. *Journal of Neuroscience, 24*(49), 11017–11022. http://dx.doi.org/10.1523/JNEUROSCI.3321-04.2004.

Hoppner, J., Broese, T., Wendler, L., Berger, C., & Thome, J. (2011). Repetitive transcranial magnetic stimulation (rTMS) for treatment of alcohol dependence. *World Journal of Biological Psychiatry, 12*(Suppl. 1), 57–62. http://dx.doi.org/10.3109/15622975.2011.598383.

Huang, Y. Z., Edwards, M. J., Rounis, E., Bhatia, K. P., & Rothwell, J. C. (2005). Theta burst stimulation of the human motor cortex. *Neuron, 45*(2), 201–206. http://dx.doi.org/10.1016/j.neuron.2004.12.033.

Ide, J. S., Zhang, S., Hu, S., Sinha, R., Mazure, C. M., & Li, C. S. (2014). Cerebral gray matter volumes and low-frequency fluctuation of BOLD signals in cocaine dependence: Duration of use and gender difference. *Drug and Alcohol Dependence, 134*, 51–62. http://dx.doi.org/10.1016/j.drugalcdep.2013.09.004.

Jacobsen, L. K., Giedd, J. N., Gottschalk, C., Kosten, T. R., & Krystal, J. H. (2001). Quantitative morphology of the caudate and putamen in patients with cocaine dependence. *The American Journal of Psychiatry, 158*(3), 486–489.

Jia, Z., Worhunsky, P. D., Carroll, K. M., Rounsaville, B. J., Stevens, M. C., Pearlson, G. D., & Potenza, M. N. (2011). An initial study of neural responses to monetary incentives as related to treatment outcome in cocaine dependence. *Biological Psychiatry, 70*(6), 553–560. http://dx.doi.org/10.1016/j.biopsych.2011.05.008.

Kaufman, J. N., Ross, T. J., Stein, E. A., & Garavan, H. (2003). Cingulate hypoactivity in cocaine users during a GO-NOGO task as revealed by event-related functional magnetic resonance imaging. *Journal of Neuroscience, 23*(21), 7839–7843.

Kelly, C., Zuo, X. N., Gotimer, K., Cox, C. L., Lynch, L., Brock, D., … Milham, M. P. (2011). Reduced interhemispheric resting state functional connectivity in cocaine addiction. *Biological Psychiatry, 69*(7), 684–692. http://dx.doi.org/10.1016/j.biopsych.2010.11.022.

Kennedy, A. P., Gross, R. E., Ely, T., Drexler, K. P., & Kilts, C. D. (2014). Clinical correlates of attentional bias to drug cues associated with cocaine dependence. *American Journal on Addictions, 23*(5), 478–484. http://dx.doi.org/10.1111/j.1521-0391.2014.12134.x.

Kilts, C. D., Gross, R. E., Ely, T. D., & Drexler, K. P. (2004). The neural correlates of cue-induced craving in cocaine-dependent women. *The American Journal of Psychiatry, 161*(2), 233–241.

Kilts, C. D., Schweitzer, J. B., Quinn, C. K., Gross, R. E., Faber, T. L., Muhammad, F., … Drexler, K. P. (2001). Neural activity related to drug craving in cocaine addiction. *Archives of General Psychiatry, 58*(4), 334–341.

Knutson, B., Westdorp, A., Kaiser, E., & Hommer, D. (2000). FMRI visualization of brain activity during a monetary incentive delay task. *Neuroimage, 12*(1), 20–27. http://dx.doi.org/10.1006/nimg.2000.0593.

Kosten, T. R., Scanley, B. E., Tucker, K. A., Oliveto, A., Prince, C., Sinha, R., … Wexler, B. E. (2006). Cue-induced brain activity changes and relapse in cocaine-dependent patients. *Neuropsychopharmacology, 31*(3), 644–650. http://dx.doi.org/10.1038/sj.npp.1300851.

Krawczyk, D. C. (2002). Contributions of the prefrontal cortex to the neural basis of human decision making. *Neuroscience & Biobehavioral Reviews, 26*(6), 631–664.

Kringelbach, M. L., & Rolls, E. T. (2004). The functional neuroanatomy of the human orbitofrontal cortex: Evidence from neuroimaging and neuropsychology. *Progress in Neurobiology*, *72*(5), 341–372. http://dx.doi.org/10.1016/j.pneurobio.2004.03.006.

Kubler, A., Murphy, K., & Garavan, H. (2005). Cocaine dependence and attention switching within and between verbal and visuospatial working memory. *European Journal of Neuroscience*, *21*(7), 1984–1992. http://dx.doi.org/10.1111/j.1460-9568.2005.04027.x.

Kufahl, P. R., Li, Z., Risinger, R. C., Rainey, C. J., Wu, G., Bloom, A. S., & Li, S. J. (2005). Neural responses to acute cocaine administration in the human brain detected by fMRI. *Neuroimage*, *28*(4), 904–914. http://dx.doi.org/10.1016/j.neuroimage.2005.06.039.

Li, X., Hartwell, K. J., Owens, M., Lematty, T., Borckardt, J. J., Hanlon, C. A., … George, M. S. (2013). Repetitive transcranial magnetic stimulation of the dorsolateral prefrontal cortex reduces nicotine cue craving. *Biological Psychiatry*, *73*(8), 714–720. http://dx.doi.org/10.1016/j.biopsych.2013.01.003.

London, E. D., Cascella, N. G., Wong, D. F., Phillips, R. L., Dannals, R. F., Links, J. M., … Wagner, H. N., Jr. (1990). Cocaine-induced reduction of glucose utilization in human brain. A study using positron emission tomography and [fluorine 18]-fluorodeoxyglucose. *Archives of General Psychiatry*, *47*(6), 567–574.

Luo, X., Zhang, S., Hu, S., Bednarski, S. R., Erdman, E., Farr, O. M., … Chiang-shan, R. L. (2013). Error processing and gender-shared and-specific neural predictors of relapse in cocaine dependence. *Brain*, *136*(4), 1231–1244.

Ma, N., Liu, Y., Li, N., Wang, C. X., Zhang, H., Jiang, X. F., … Zhang, D. R. (2010). Addiction related alteration in resting-state brain connectivity. *Neuroimage*, *49*(1), 738–744. http://dx.doi.org/10.1016/j.neuroimage.2009.08.037.

Maas, L. C., Lukas, S. E., Kaufman, M. J., Weiss, R. D., Daniels, S. L., Rogers, V. W., … Renshaw, P. F. (1998). Functional magnetic resonance imaging of human brain activation during cue-induced cocaine craving. *The American Journal of Psychiatry*, *155*(1), 124–126.

Makris, N., Gasic, G. P., Kennedy, D. N., Hodge, S. M., Kaiser, J. R., Lee, M. J., … Breiter, H. C. (2008). Cortical thickness abnormalities in cocaine addiction—A reflection of both drug use and a pre-existing disposition to drug abuse? *Neuron*, *60*(1), 174–188. http://dx.doi.org/10.1016/j.neuron.2008.08.011.

Makris, N., Gasic, G. P., Seidman, L. J., Goldstein, J. M., Gastfriend, D. R., Elman, I., … Breiter, H. C. (2004). Decreased absolute amygdala volume in cocaine addicts. *Neuron*, *44*(4), 729–740. http://dx.doi.org/10.1016/j.neuron.2004.10.027.

Marhe, R., Luijten, M., van de Wetering, B. J., Smits, M., & Franken, I. H. (2013). Individual differences in anterior cingulate activation associated with attentional bias predict cocaine use after treatment. *Neuropsychopharmacology*, *38*(6), 1085–1093.

Matochik, J. A., London, E. D., Eldreth, D. A., Cadet, J. L., & Bolla, K. I. (2003). Frontal cortical tissue composition in abstinent cocaine abusers: A magnetic resonance imaging study. *Neuroimage*, *19*(3), 1095–1102.

McHugh, M. J., Demers, C. H., Braud, J., Briggs, R., Adinoff, B., & Stein, E. A. (2013). Striatal-insula circuits in cocaine addiction: Implications for impulsivity and relapse risk. *American Journal of Drug and Alcohol Abuse*, *39*(6), 424–432. http://dx.doi.org/10.3109/00952990.2013.847446.

McHugh, M. J., Demers, C. H., Salmeron, B. J., Devous, M. D., Sr., Stein, E. A., & Adinoff, B. (2014). Cortico-amygdala coupling as a marker of early relapse risk in cocaine-addicted individuals. *Front Psychiatry*, *5*, 16. http://dx.doi.org/10.3389/fpsyt.2014.00016.

Mei, S., Xu, J., Carroll, K. M., & Potenza, M. N. (2015). Self-reported impulsivity is negatively correlated with amygdala volumes in cocaine dependence. *Psychiatry Research*, *233*(2), 212–217. http://dx.doi.org/10.1016/j.pscychresns.2015.07.013.

Mishra, B. R., Nizamie, S. H., Das, B., & Praharaj, S. K. (2010). Efficacy of repetitive transcranial magnetic stimulation in alcohol dependence: A sham-controlled study. *Addiction*, *105*(1), 49–55. http://dx.doi.org/10.1111/j.1360-0443.2009.02777.x.

Mitchell, M. R., Balodis, I. M., Devito, E. E., Lacadie, C. M., Yeston, J., Scheinost, D., … Potenza, M. N. (2013). A preliminary investigation of Stroop-related intrinsic connectivity in cocaine dependence: Associations with treatment outcomes. *American Journal of Drug and Alcohol Abuse*, *39*(6), 392–402. http://dx.doi.org/10.3109/00952990.2013.841711.

Moeller, F. G., Dougherty, D. M., Barratt, E. S., Schmitz, J. M., Swann, A. C., & Grabowski, J. (2001). The impact of impulsivity on cocaine use and retention in treatment. *Journal of Substance Abuse Treatment*, *21*(4), 193–198. http://dx.doi.org/10.1016/s0740-5472(01)00202-1.

Moeller, F. G., Steinberg, J. L., Schmitz, J. M., Ma, L., Liu, S., Kjome, K. L., … Narayana, P. A. (2010). Working memory fMRI activation in cocaine-dependent subjects: Association with treatment response. *Psychiatry Research*, *181*(3), 174–182. http://dx.doi.org/10.1016/j.pscychresns.2009.11.003.

Moeller, S. J., Tomasi, D., Honorio, J., Volkow, N. D., & Goldstein, R. Z. (2012). Dopaminergic involvement during mental fatigue in health and cocaine addiction. *Translational Psychiatry*, *2*, e176. http://dx.doi.org/10.1038/tp.2012.110.

Neto, L. L., Oliveira, E., Correia, F., & Ferreira, A. G. (2008). The human nucleus accumbens: Where is it? A stereotactic, anatomical and magnetic resonance imaging study. *Neuromodulation*, *11*(1), 13–22. http://dx.doi.org/10.1111/j.1525-1403.2007.00138.x.

Noonan, M. A., Bulin, S. E., Fuller, D. C., & Eisch, A. J. (2010). Reduction of adult hippocampal neurogenesis confers vulnerability in an animal model of cocaine addiction. *Journal of Neuroscience*, *30*(1), 304–315. http://dx.doi.org/10.1523/JNEUROSCI.4256-09.2010.

O'Neill, J., Cardenas, V. A., & Meyerhoff, D. J. (2001). Separate and interactive effects of cocaine and alcohol dependence on brain structures and metabolites: Quantitative MRI and proton MR spectroscopic imaging. *Addiction Biology*, *6*(4), 347–361. http://dx.doi.org/10.1080/13556210020077073.

Pallasch, T. J., & Joseph, C. E. (1987). Oral manifestations of drug abuse. *Journal of Psychoactive Drugs*, *19*(4), 375–377. http://dx.doi.org/10.1080/02791072.1987.10472425.

Parvaz M.A., Moeller S.J., d'Oleire Uquillas F., Pflumm A., Maloney T., Alia-Klein N., & Goldstein R.Z. (2016). Prefrontal gray matter volume recovery in treatment-seeking cocaine-addicted individuals: A longitudinal study, *Addiction Biology*, in press, http://dx.doi.org/10.1111/adb.12403.

Politi, E., Fauci, E., Santoro, A., & Smeraldi, E. (2008). Daily sessions of transcranial magnetic stimulation to the left prefrontal cortex gradually reduce cocaine craving. *American Journal on Addictions*, *17*(4), 345–346. http://dx.doi.org/10.1080/10550490802139283.

Porrino, L. J., Lyons, D., Smith, H. R., Daunais, J. B., & Nader, M. A. (2004). Cocaine self-administration produces a progressive involvement of limbic, association, and sensorimotor striatal domains. *Journal of Neuroscience*, *24*(14), 3554–3562. http://dx.doi.org/10.1523/JNEUROSCI.5578-03.2004.

Pripfl, J., Tomova, L., Riecansky, I., & Lamm, C. (2014). Transcranial magnetic stimulation of the left dorsolateral prefrontal cortex decreases cue-induced nicotine craving and EEG delta power. *Brain Stimulation*, 7(2), 226–233. http://dx.doi.org/10.1016/j.brs.2013.11.003.

Prisciandaro, J. J., Myrick, H., Henderson, S., McRae-Clark, A. L., & Brady, K. T. (2013). Prospective associations between brain activation to cocaine and no-go cues and cocaine relapse. *Drug and Alcohol Dependence*, *131*(1–2), 44–49. http://dx.doi.org/10.1016/j.drugalcdep.2013.04.008.

Risinger, R. C., Salmeron, B. J., Ross, T. J., Amen, S. L., Sanfilipo, M., Hoffmann, R. G., ... Stein, E. A. (2005). Neural correlates of high and craving during cocaine self-administration using BOLD fMRI. *Neuroimage*, *26*(4), 1097–1108. http://dx.doi.org/10.1016/j.neuroimage.2005.03.030.

Rogers, J. L., & See, R. E. (2007). Selective inactivation of the ventral hippocampus attenuates cue-induced and cocaine-primed reinstatement of drug-seeking in rats. *Neurobiology of Learning and Memory*, *87*(4), 688–692. http://dx.doi.org/10.1016/j.nlm.2007.01.003.

See, R. E. (2005). Neural substrates of cocaine-cue associations that trigger relapse. *European Journal of Pharmacology*, *526*(1–3), 140–146. http://dx.doi.org/10.1016/j.ejphar.2005.09.034.

Sim, M. E., Lyoo, I. K., Streeter, C. C., Covell, J., Sarid-Segal, O., Ciraulo, D. A., ... Renshaw, P. F. (2007). Cerebellar gray matter volume correlates with duration of cocaine use in cocaine-dependent subjects. *Neuropsychopharmacology*, *32*(10), 2229–2237. http://dx.doi.org/10.1038/sj.npp.1301346.

Singer, T., Critchley, H. D., & Preuschoff, K. (2009). A common role of insula in feelings, empathy and uncertainty. *Trends in Cognitive Science*, *13*(8), 334–340. http://dx.doi.org/10.1016/j.tics.2009.05.001.

Sinha, R., Lacadie, C., Skudlarski, P., Fulbright, R. K., Rounsaville, B. J., Kosten, T. R., & Wexler, B. E. (2005). Neural activity associated with stress-induced cocaine craving: A functional magnetic resonance imaging study. *Psychopharmacology*, *183*(2), 171–180. http://dx.doi.org/10.1007/s00213-005-0147-8.

Stagg, C. J., Wylezinska, M., Matthews, P. M., Johansen-Berg, H., Jezzard, P., Rothwell, J. C., & Bestmann, S. (2009). Neurochemical effects of theta burst stimulation as assessed by magnetic resonance spectroscopy. *Journal of Neurophysiology*, *101*(6), 2872–2877. http://dx.doi.org/10.1152/jn.91060.2008.

Strafella, A. P., Paus, T., Barrett, J., & Dagher, A. (2001). Repetitive transcranial magnetic stimulation of the human prefrontal cortex induces dopamine release in the caudate nucleus. *Journal of Neuroscience*, *21*(15), RC157.

Streeter, C. C., Terhune, D. B., Whitfield, T. H., Gruber, S., Sarid-Segal, O., Silveri, M. M., ... Yurgelun-Todd, D. A. (2008). Performance on the Stroop predicts treatment compliance in cocaine-dependent individuals. *Neuropsychopharmacology*, *33*(4), 827–836. http://dx.doi.org/10.1038/sj.npp.1301465.

Thickbroom, G. W. (2007). Transcranial magnetic stimulation and synaptic plasticity: Experimental framework and human models. *Experimental Brain Research*, *180*(4), 583–593. http://dx.doi.org/10.1007/s00221-007-0991-3.

Tomasi, D., Goldstein, R. Z., Telang, F., Maloney, T., Alia-Klein, N., Caparelli, E. C., & Volkow, N. D. (2007a). Thalamo-cortical dysfunction in cocaine abusers: Implications in attention and perception. *Psychiatry Research*, *155*(3), 189–201. http://dx.doi.org/10.1016/j.pscychresns.2007.03.002.

Tomasi, D., Goldstein, R. Z., Telang, F., Maloney, T., Alia-Klein, N., Caparelli, E. C., & Volkow, N. D. (2007b). Widespread disruption in brain activation patterns to a working memory task during cocaine abstinence. *Brain Research*, *1171*, 83–92. http://dx.doi.org/10.1016/j.brainres.2007.06.102.

Tseng, W., Sutter, M. E., & Albertson, T. E. (2014). Stimulants and the lung: Review of literature. *Clinical Reviews in Allergy & Immunology*, *46*(1), 82–100. http://dx.doi.org/10.1007/s12016-013-8376-9.

Verdejo-García, A., Bechara, A., Recknor, E. C., & Pérez-García, M. (2006). Executive dysfunction in substance dependent individuals during drug use and abstinence: An examination of the behavioral, cognitive and emotional correlates of addiction. *Journal of the International Neuropsychological Society*, *12*(3), 405–415. http://dx.doi.org/10.1017/s1355617706060486.

Vogt, B. A., Vogt, L., & Laureys, S. (2006). Cytology and functionally correlated circuits of human posterior cingulate areas. *Neuroimage, 29*(2), 452–466. http://dx.doi.org/10.1016/j.neuroimage.2005.07.048.

Volkow, N. D., & Fowler, J. S. (2000). Addiction, a disease of compulsion and drive: Involvement of the orbitofrontal cortex. *Cerebral Cortex, 10*(3), 318–325.

Volkow, N. D., Fowler, J. S., Wang, G. J., Hitzemann, R., Logan, J., Schlyer, D. J., … Wolf, A. P. (1993). Decreased dopamine D2 receptor availability is associated with reduced frontal metabolism in cocaine abusers. *Synapse, 14*(2), 169–177. http://dx.doi.org/10.1002/syn.890140210.

Volkow, N. D., Fowler, J. S., Wolf, A. P., Hitzemann, R., Dewey, S., Bendriem, B., … Hoff, A. (1991). Changes in brain glucose metabolism in cocaine dependence and withdrawal. *The American Journal of Psychiatry, 148*(5), 621–626.

Volkow, N. D., Hitzemann, R., Wang, G. J., Fowler, J. S., Wolf, A. P., Dewey, S. L., & Handlesman, L. (1992). Long-term frontal brain metabolic changes in cocaine abusers. *Synapse, 11*(3), 184–190. http://dx.doi.org/10.1002/syn.890110303.

Volkow, N. D., Wang, G. J., Fowler, J. S., Tomasi, D., & Telang, F. (2011). Addiction: Beyond dopamine reward circuitry. *Proceedings of the National Academy of Sciences of the United States of America, 108*(37), 15037–15042. http://dx.doi.org/10.1073/pnas.1010654108.

Volkow, N. D., Wang, G. J., Ma, Y., Fowler, J. S., Wong, C., Ding, Y. S., … Kalivas, P. (2005). Activation of orbital and medial prefrontal cortex by methylphenidate in cocaine-addicted subjects but not in controls: Relevance to addiction. *Journal of Neuroscience, 25*(15), 3932–3939. http://dx.doi.org/10.1523/JNEUROSCI.0433-05.2005.

Wilcox, C. E., Teshiba, T. M., Merideth, F., Ling, J., & Mayer, A. R. (2011). Enhanced cue reactivity and fronto-striatal functional connectivity in cocaine use disorders. *Drug and Alcohol Dependence, 115*(1–2), 137–144. http://dx.doi.org/10.1016/j.drugalcdep.2011.01.009.

Wing, V. C., Barr, M. S., Wass, C. E., Lipsman, N., Lozano, A. M., Daskalakis, Z. J., & George, T. P. (2013). Brain stimulation methods to treat tobacco addiction. *Brain Stimulation, 6*(3), 221–230. http://dx.doi.org/10.1016/j.brs.2012.06.008.

Wong, D. F., Kuwabara, H., Schretlen, D. J., Bonson, K. R., Zhou, Y., Nandi, A., … London, E. D. (2006). Increased occupancy of dopamine receptors in human striatum during cue-elicited cocaine craving. *Neuropsychopharmacology, 31*(12), 2716–2727. http://dx.doi.org/10.1038/sj.npp.1301194.

Worhunsky, P. D., Stevens, M. C., Carroll, K. M., Rounsaville, B. J., Calhoun, V. D., Pearlson, G. D., & Potenza, M. N. (2013). Functional brain networks associated with cognitive control, cocaine dependence, and treatment outcome. *Psychology of Addictive Behaviors, 27*(2), 477–488. http://dx.doi.org/10.1037/a0029092.

Xu, J., Kober, H., Wang, X., DeVito, E. E., Carroll, K. M., & Potenza, M. N. (2014). Hippocampal volume mediates the relationship between measures of pre-treatment cocaine use and within-treatment cocaine abstinence. *Drug and Alcohol Dependence, 143*, 74–80. http://dx.doi.org/10.1016/j.drugalcdep.2014.07.007.

Yu, C., Zhou, Y., Liu, Y., Jiang, T., Dong, H., Zhang, Y., & Walter, M. (2011). Functional segregation of the human cingulate cortex is confirmed by functional connectivity based neuroanatomical parcellation. *Neuroimage, 54*(4), 2571–2581. http://dx.doi.org/10.1016/j.neuroimage.2010.11.018.

CHAPTER SEVEN

Treating Addiction: Perspectives from EEG and Imaging Studies on Psychedelics

L.F. Tófoli*[,1], D.B. de Araujo†
*School of Medical Sciences, University of Campinas, Campinas, Brazil
†Brain Institute/Hospital Universitario Onofre Lopes, UFRN, Natal, Brazil
[1]Corresponding author: e-mail address: lftofoli@gmail.com

Contents

Abstract

Despite reports of apparent benefits, social and political pressure beginning in the late 1960s effectively banned scientific inquiry into psychedelic substances. Covert examination of psychedelics persisted through the 1990s; the turn of the century and especially the past 10 years, however, has seen a resurgent interest in psychedelic substances (eg, LSD, ayahuasca, psilocybin). This chapter outlines relevant EEG and brain imaging studies evaluating the effects of psychedelics on the brain. This chapter also reviews evidence of the use of psychedelics as adjunct therapy for a number of psychiatric and addictive disorders. In particular, psychedelics appear to have efficacy in treating depression and alcohol-use disorders.

1. INTRODUCTION

Psychedelics have long been used by native cultures in various rituals (Schultes, 1979). In spite of countercultural connotations of the term

International Review of Neurobiology, Volume 129
ISSN 0074-7742
http://dx.doi.org/10.1016/bs.irn.2016.06.005

psychedelic—coined by Sir Humphrey Osmond to mean "mind manifesting" —this appellation has been carefully chosen by scientists involved in "psychedelic renaissance" studies (Sessa, 2012). The term may include substances with a number of different pharmacological profiles, including serotonin agonists, glutamatergic *N*-methyl-D-aspartate receptor antagonists, κ-opioid receptor agonists, anticholinergic agents, and cannabinoids (Szabó, Kazai, Frecska, & Brys, 2015). Depending on the drug, dose, setting, and personal predisposition, the altered state of consciousness associated with psychedelics often includes cognitive changes; broad perceptual changes; profound experiential changes in mood, thought, insight, and memory; and mystical and transpersonal experiences including illusions and hallucinations (Nichols, 2004).

Based on their effects, these compounds can be categorized into deliriants, dissociatives, and classic psychedelics. Deliriants, such as plant-derived scopolamine and atropine and synthetic dimenhydrinate and trihexyphenidyl, commonly involve acetylcholine antagonism and tend to induce true hallucinations, delusions, and delirium (eg, stupor, confusion, confabulation). Dissociative hallucinogens, apart from perceptual changes, invoke a sense of detachment or dissociative anesthesia, described as oneirophrenia (dreamlike mind). Mechanisms of action of dissociative hallucinogens include NMDA receptor antagonisms (eg, ketamine and phencyclidine—PCP) and κ-opioid agonism (eg, salvinorin A, the active component of *Salvia divinorum*). Ibogaine is also a NMDA receptor antagonist and considered a dissociative hallucinogen, but its pharmacodynamics are complex and may include serotonin and opioid systems (Popik, Layer, & Skolnick, 1995). This chapter will focus on the properties of classic or serotonergic psychedelics. Methylenedioxymethamphetamine (MDMA, also known as "ecstasy" or "molly") and other phenethylamines with empathogenic properties are sometimes considered psychedelics, since they also act on serotonin receptors but because they also have amphetamine-like characteristics and are rarely hallucinogenic in the classical sense, they will not be included herein.

Based on their chemical profiles, classic psychedelics can be classified into three main categories: tryptamines, such as psilocybin, found in "magic mushrooms," and *N*,*N*-dimethyltryptamine (DMT); phenethylamines, such as mescaline and dl-2,5-dimethoxy-4-methylamphetamine (DOM); and lysergamides, such as lysergic acid diethylamide (LSD), with both tryptamine and phenethylamine properties, have efficacy primarily as partial agonists at serotonin $5HT_{2A}$ receptors.

Classic psychedelics modulate serotonin ($5HT_{2A}$) receptors, although recent work suggests involvement of sigma-1 receptors (Fontanilla et al., 2009). They include psilocybin, ayahuasca, mescaline, and LSD, which have very low addictive potential (Shmulewitz, Greene, & Hasin, 2015) and increasing evidence suggests that they may be an alternative tool in the treatment of addiction (Bogenschutz, 2013; Bogenschutz et al., 2015; Bogenschutz & Johnson, 2016; Bogenschutz & Pommy, 2012; Dakwar, Levin, Foltin, Nunes, & Hart, 2014; Dyck, 2009; Liester & Prickett, 2012; Mangini, 1998; Ross, 2012; Sewell, Halpern, & Pope, 2006; Vollenweider & Kometer, 2010; Winkelman, 2014).

This chapter has two aims. The first aim is to present the available studies that have used electroencephalography (EEG), magnetoencephalography (MEG), positron emission tomography (PET), single-photon emission computed tomography (SPECT), or functional magnetic resonance imaging (fMRI) to investigate the human brain under the influence of classic psychedelics. The second aim is to discuss their use as therapeutic options to treat drug addiction.

2. BRAIN RESEARCH STUDIES OF CLASSIC PSYCHEDELICS

Knowledge about plants and substances with psychedelic properties is not new to modern science: mescaline was isolated by Arthur Heffter in the late 19th century, and the effects of LSD were identified by Albert Hofmann in 1943 (Stafford, 1992). Nevertheless, our knowledge about the mechanisms of action of these substances remains superficial, in part due to the research embargo this field has been subjected for many decades, at least since the end of the 1960s, as a result of the "war on drugs" (Oram, 2014; Rowe, 2006).

While scientific studies using psilocybin have been taking place since the end of the 20th century (Carhart-Harris, Bolstridge, et al., 2016; Carhart-Harris, Erritzoe, et al., 2012; Carhart-Harris et al., 2011; Gouzoulis-Mayfrank, Schreckenberger, et al., 1999; Gouzoulis-Mayfrank, Thelen, et al., 1999; Kraehenmann et al., 2015; Palhano-Fontes et al., 2015), LSD, the most paradigmatic of all psychedelics, has only recently reentered the scope of modern science (Gasser et al.,

2014). This is also true for the evaluation of psychedelics using modern neuroimaging techniques: in spite of the rapid proliferation of MRI-based psychiatric, pharmacological, and psychological studies, relatively few publications have used MRI to assess the effects of psychedelics on the human brain.

2.1 Ayahuasca

Ayahuasca (the "vine of the spirits" in Quechua) is a psychedelic brew traditionally used by Amerindians that reached Brazilian urban centers around 1930, where it has since been used as a sacrament in syncretic churches such as the Santo Daime, the União do Vegetal (UDV), and Barquinha. More recently, the use of ayahuasca has expanded to the United States and Europe (Labate & Cavnar, 2011). There are numerous recipes that may be used to prepare ayahuasca, although it is most frequently produced by the decoction of the bark of a liana named *Banisteriopsis caapi* (*B. caapi*) with the leaves of a DMT-containing plant, *Psychotria viridis* (Ott, 1994). Indigenous traditions consider the *B. caapi* vine to be the main ingredient of ayahuasca and name the brew after the native species (eg, ayahuasca, natem, yagé, nixi pae). In research studies, it is important to keep in mind the potential diversity of components of ayahuasca (Brierley & Davidson, 2012), since it has come from a number of different plants and cultivars collected at different times.

Compared to other psychedelics, the pharmacology of ayahuasca is particularly complex. DMT is mostly inactive when taken orally due to the presence of monoamine oxidase (MAO) enzymes in the gut. However, *B. caapi* is rich in β-carboline alkaloids (eg, harmine and harmaline), which are reversible MAO inhibitors. The constituents of ayahuasca therefore protect DMT from degradation, allowing its access to the central nervous system (McKenna, 2004). Also, MAO inhibition likely has direct impact on the brain, as these enzymes protect other monoamines, such as serotonin, dopamine, and norepinephrine, from oxidative deamination. Furthermore, β-carbolines may have psychoactive properties independent of MAO inhibition. For example, another component of ayahuasca, tetrahydroharmine (THH), is a serotonin reuptake inhibitor (SSRI). It is still in dispute to what extent harmine, harmaline, and THH have independent psychedelic effects (Naranjo, 1987; Ott, 1994; Shulgin, 1980).

The acute effects of ayahuasca begin approximately 30–40 min after oral intake, and last up to 4 h. Autonomic responses include increases in cardiac and respiratory rates, blood pressure, temperature, and pupil diameter

(Callaway et al., 1996; Riba et al., 2003). Ayahuasca effects also include changes in perception, altered spatiotemporal scaling, enhanced visual imagery (especially with eyes closed), increased introspection, changes in mood, and the memories with high emotional salience (Shanon, 2003).

Results of several research studies using ayahuasca are presented in Table 1. The first EEG study using ayahuasca was conducted in 11 members of the Santo Daime church in a ritual setting. Increased gamma power was observed in left occipital–temporal–parietal electrodes, during the eyes-closed condition. With eyes open, significant increased gamma power was restricted to occipital electrodes (Don et al., 1998). In another EEG study of 12 experienced individuals after three doses, ayahuasca increased power of both alpha and theta bands when compared to baseline. The strongest increase of alpha activity was observed in occipital electrodes; alpha was unchanged in the frontal electrodes and theta power significantly increased in both occipital and frontal areas (Hoffman et al., 2001).

The first set of well-controlled experiments was performed with a low (0.6 mg/kg of DMT) and high (0.85 mg/kg of DMT) dose of encapsulated, freeze-dried ayahuasca administered to 18 volunteers with previous psychedelic experience, in a double-blind crossover, placebo-controlled design. Absolute power decreased in all frequency bands, most prominently in theta; relative power of delta decreased. There was also an increase in beta power. Observed EEG changes began 15–30 min after ayahuasca intake, reached a peak between 45 and 120 min, and thereafter decreased to baseline 4–6 h after administration (Barbanoj et al., 2008; Riba et al., 2004, 2002). The spatial distribution of brain electrical activity was investigated using low-resolution electromagnetic tomography (LORETA) and a high dose (ie, 0.85 mg/kg of DMT) compared to placebo. Statistically significant differences, found at 60 and 90 min after ayahuasca intake, showed decreases in the alpha, delta, theta, and beta bands. Analysis with LORETA indicated that power decreases in delta, alpha, and beta bands occurred in the temporo-parieto-occipital junction, while theta decrease was localized to temporomedial and frontomedial regions (Riba et al., 2004).

To investigate the impact of daytime ayahuasca consumption on sleep, as measured by polysomnography (Barbanoj et al., 2008), freeze-dried ayahuasca (equivalent to 1 mg/kg of DMT), and an active placebo of D-amphetamine (20 mg) were administered to 22 healthy male volunteers in a randomized, double-blind, placebo-controlled, crossover design. Subjects ingested ayahuasca or amphetamine during the day, and sleep was evaluated the following night. In contrast with D-amphetamine, ayahuasca did not

Table 1 EEG and Imaging Studies with Ayahuasca

Method	Subjects	Dose: Presentation	Dose: DMT	Dose: HRM	Dose: HRL	Dose: THH	Design	Start of Acquisition After Dosing	Results	Reference(s)
EEG	11 Santo Daime members	Liquid Average dose (75 mL)	0.546 mg/mL 41 mg	0.741 mg/mL 55.6 mg	0.061 mg/mL 4.6 mg	0.585 mg/mL 43.9 mg	Religious ritual setting, single dose, no placebo	45–60 min	Increased power in higher frequencies (36–44 Hz) in left occipital–temporal–parietal scalp electrodes with eyes closed. Effect extended to most of the posterior scalp with eyes open. Tendencies toward decrease in power of slow (theta and alpha) waves and increases in beta	Don et al. (1998)
EEG	12 Healthy volunteers	Not quantified					Shamanic setting, acquisition after three doses, no placebo	1–2 h After the third dose (4–6 h after the first one)	Strong increases in alpha and theta mean amplitudes. Beta amplitudes unchanged. Strongest increases of alpha activity in occipital lobes, unchanged in the frontal lobes. Theta amplitudes increased in all parts of the brain, except for the right temporal and posttemporal areas	Hoffman, Hesselink, and Silveira-Barbosa (2001)
Topographic EEG	18 Healthy volunteers	Original liquid Low dose (dried) High dose (dried)	0.53 mg/mL 0.6 mg/kg 0.85 mg/kg	0.90 mg/mL 1.02 mg/kg 1.44 mg/kg	0.06 mg/mL 0.07 mg/kg 0.1 mg/kg	0.72 mg/mL 0.82 mg/kg 1.15 mg/kg	Double-blind crossover design with placebo and two doses (low and high) of freeze-dried ayahuasca	"Regular intervals"	Absolute power decreased in all frequency bands, most prominently in theta. Relative power decreased in delta and theta and increased in alpha and beta (especially faster beta-3 and beta-4). Findings were dose dependent	Riba et al. (2002)
EEG/LORETA								30, 60, 90, 120, 180, 360, and 480 min	Only the high dose was assessed. Differences found at 60 and 90 min of intake. Power density decreased in alpha-2, delta, theta, and beta-1. Power decreases in delta, alpha-2, and beta-1 detected over temporo-parieto-occipital junction. Theta power reductions registered in temporomedial and frontomedial regions	Riba, Anderer, Jane, Saletu, and Barbanoj (2004)
EEG/PSG	22 Male healthy volunteers	Freeze dried	1.0 mg/kg	1.70 mg/kg	0.11 mg/kg	1.36 mg/kg	Double-blind crossover design; administration of ayahuasca, D-amphetamine (20 mg) and placebo	9 h	No deterioration of sleep quality or PSG disruptions of sleep initiation or maintenance with ayahuasca, different from D-amphetamine. Both ayahuasca and D-amphetamine decreased REM, with a trend increase in REM sleep onset latency. While D-amphetamine decreased slow-wave sleep (SWS) power in the first nigh cycle, the opposite happened with ayahuasca	Barbanoj et al. (2008)
Topographic EEG	20 Healthy volunteers	Liquid	0.328 mg/mL 1.39 mg/kg	1.08 mg/mL 4.58 mg/kg	0.18 mg/mL 0.75 mg/kg	1.28 mg/mL 5.43 mg/kg	Open-label, pre-, and postayahuasca comparison	25, 50, 75, 100, and 125 min	First phase (from 50 min, associated with DMT and harmine plasma levels): reduced power in alpha, mostly at the left parieto-occipital cortex. Second phase (between 75 and 125 min,	Schenberg et al. (2015)

									correlated with harmaline and THH levels): increased in slow-gamma power at left centro-parieto-occipital, left frontotemporal, and right frontal cortices, and of fast-gamma at left centro-parieto-occipital, left frontotemporal, right frontal, and right parieto-occipital cortices	
SPECT	15 Healthy male volunteers	Original liquid Freeze dried	0.53 mg/mL 1.0 mg/kg	0.90 mg/mL 1.70 mg/kg	0.06 mg/mL 0.11 mg/kg	0.72 mg/mL 1.36 mg/kg	Double-blind, placebo controlled	100–110 min	Increased blood perfusion observed bilaterally in the anterior insula (more intense in the right hemisphere), and right anterior cingulate/frontomedial cortex increased blood flow in the left amygdala/parahippocampal gyrus	Riba et al. (2006)
SPECT	17 Patients with recurrent depression	Liquid	0.8 mg/mL 1.76 mg/kg	0.21 mg/mL 0.46 mg/kg	Not detected	Not informed	Open-label, single dose, no placebo	8 h	Increases in blood perfusion in the left nucleus accumbens, right insula, and left subgenual area	Sanches et al. (2016)
fMRI/BOLD	9 Healthy members of Santo Daime						Open-label, single dose, no placebo, before/after intake comparisons	40 min	Acquisition made during a mental imagery task with eyes open and closed. Robust increases in the activation of several occipital, temporal, and frontal areas during mental imagery task with eyes closed, but not with eyes open. Potentiated activity of parahippocampal gyrus, right fusiform, and right middle occipital gyrus. Positive modulation of middle and superior frontal gyrus	de Araujo et al. (2012)
fMRI								Resting state	Decreased activity through most parts of the default mode network, including its most consistent hubs: the posterior cingulate cortex (PCC)/precuneus and the medial prefrontal cortex. Functional connectivity within the PCC/precuneus was decreased. No decrease in orthogonality (enhanced connectivity) between the default mode and the task-positive networks	Palhano-Fontes et al. (2015)
sMRI	22 Regular ayahuasca users and 22 controls	Ayahuasca users were members of Santo Daime; average lifetime use: 123 times (range: 50–352)					Case-control study	Does not apply	Differences from controls were found in midline brain structures. With a thinning in the posterior cingulate cortex of ayahuasca users. PCC cortical thickness was inversely correlated with intensity and duration of prior ayahuasca use and with self-transcendence scores	Bouso, Palhano-Fontes, Rodríguez-Fornells, et al. (2015)

Note: BOLD, blood-oxygen-level-dependent contrast imaging; *DMT*, *N,N*-dimethyltryptamine; *EEG*, electroencephalography; *fMRI*, functional magnetic resonance imaging; *HRM*, harmine; *HRL*, harmaline; *LORETA*, low-resolution electromagnetic tomography; *PCC*, posterior cingulate cortex; *SPECT*, single-photon emission computed tomography; *sMRI*, structural magnetic resonance imaging; *THH*, tetrahydroharmine.

induce any subjectively perceived deterioration of sleep quality or disruptions of sleep initiation and/or maintenance. Both ayahuasca and D-amphetamine inhibited rapid eye movement (REM) sleep, decreasing its duration in absolute values and as a percentage of total sleep time, and showed a trend to increase REM onset. On the other hand, D-amphetamine decreased slow-wave sleep (SWS) power, while ayahuasca increased SWS power (Barbanoj et al., 2008).

The most recently published EEG study on ayahuasca investigated the relationship between temporal changes in EEG measures with serum concentrations of the main components of ayahuasca. Ayahuasca, donated by UDV, was given *in natura* to 20 individuals with previous experience. There was no blinding or placebo control. A biphasic effect of ayahuasca was found. The first phase showed reduced alpha power, 50 min after ingestion; the second phase was characterized by an increase in slow- and fast-gamma (30–50 and 50–100 Hz, respectively) power 75 and 125 min after ingestion. Alpha power decrease was most evident on the left parieto-occipital cortex. Slow-gamma increases were localized to the left centro-parieto-occipital, left frontotemporal, and right frontal cortices, while the fast-gamma increases were found on the left centro-parieto-occipital, left frontotemporal, right frontal, and right parieto-occipital cortices. These effects were significantly associated with circulating levels of DMT, harmine, harmaline, THH, and some of their metabolites (Schenberg et al., 2015).

A SPECT study using freeze-dried ayahuasca in a placebo-controlled design evaluated healthy male volunteers ($n = 15$) with previous psychedelic experience, scanned 100–110 min after ayahuasca administration. Significantly increased cerebral blood flow (CBF) was observed bilaterally in the anterior insula, asymmetric to the right hemisphere, in the right anterior cingulate cortex (ACC)/frontomedial cortex, and in the left amygdala/parahippocampal gyrus (Riba et al., 2006).

fMRI has also been used to investigate the acute effects of ayahuasca (de Araujo et al., 2012; Palhano-Fontes et al., 2015). fMRI was acquired before and after (40 min) ayahuasca, from nine members of the Santo Daime church, who performed a visual perception and a mental imagery task. This study suggests that ayahuasca selectively increases the activity of the primary and higher visual cortices (BA17, 18, and 19), the parahippocampal gyrus (BA30), and the right fusiform gyrus (BA37). A positive modulation was also found in the frontopolar cortex (BA10) (de Araujo et al., 2012). In another fMRI study, ayahuasca significantly decreased the activity in many regions of the Default Mode Network (DMN), particularly the posterior cingulate cortex (PCC)/precuneus. Also, decreased functional connectivity between the PCC/precuneus and other regions was observed during the effects of ayahuasca (Palhano-Fontes et al., 2015). The DMN is a set of brain regions with higher activity at rest (eyes-closed) relative to externally oriented tasks and has been associated with a variety of mental states, including mind wandering and rumination (Hamilton, Farmer, Fogelman, & Gotlib, 2015; Tops, Boksem, Quirin, IJzerman, & Koole, 2014).

2.2 Psilocybin

Psilocybin, an indolealkylamine and tryptamine, is the main active ingredient of the group of fungi known as "magic mushrooms." Psilocybin is a prodrug, that is, a substance that is metabolized after administration to become pharmacologically active as psilocin. When given orally, psilocybin is almost entirely transformed into psilocin during first-pass liver metabolism. Intravenous administration requires conversion of psilocybin to psilocin in the kidneys, a process that may be less efficient (Hasler, Bourquin, Brenneisen, Bar, & Vollenweider, 1997; Passie, Seifert, Schneider, & Emrich, 2002). The neuropsychological effects of psilocin appear to be mediated by stimulation of serotonergic receptors, namely, subtypes $5HT_{2A}$, $5HT_{2C}$, and $5HT_{1C}$. Psilocybin is well tolerated and safe for human studies at oral doses of 8–25 mg and intravenous doses of 1–2 mg (Passie et al., 2002; Shulgin, 1980; Tylš, Páleníček, & Horáček, 2014).

Results of several research studies using psilocybin are presented in Table 2, together with the few mescaline and LSD studies available. A PET study used [^{18}F]-fluorodeoxyglucose (FDG) to assess cerebral metabolic rate of glucose utilization (MRglu) following psilocybin administration (Vollenweider et al., 1997). Ten healthy volunteers were scanned before and 90 min after receiving a single oral dose of psilocybin (15 mg to subjects $\leq$ 50 kg or 20 mg to subject $\geq$ 51 kg body weight). Psilocybin produced a global increase ($\sim$25%) of MRglu, most prominent in frontomedial and frontolateral cortices, ACC, and temporomedial cortex. Increased MRglu was also found in the basal ganglia ($\sim$19%) and in sensorimotor and occipital cortices ($\sim$14%). Significant correlations were found between "psychotic-like symptoms" and increased MRglu in the prefrontal cortex.

EEG/MEG studies with psilocybin have shown decreased parieto-occipital alpha power (Kometer, Schmidt, Jancke, & Vollenweider, 2013).

Table 2 EEG and Imaging Studies with Psilocybin, Mescaline, and LSD

Method	Subjects	Drug	Dosage	Design	Start of Acquisition After Dosing	Effects of Psychedelic Substance	References
SPECT	23 Male healthy volunteers	Mescaline (oral)	500 mg	Open design: 11 in mescaline and 12 in placebo group; ^{99m}Tc-HMPAO-assessed CBF	4½ h	Pattern of hyperfrontality with emphasis on right hemisphere in mescaline group	Hermle et al. (1992)
						Right-hemisphere lateralization only on the anterior cortical regions in mescaline group	Hermle, Gouzoulis-Mayfrank, and Spitzer (1998)
PET/MRglu	10 Healthy volunteers	Psilocybin (oral)	15 mg (subjects ≤ 50 kg) or 20 mg (≥ 51 kg)	Single-blind design (volunteers received one of three drugs); [^{18}F] FDG-assessed MRglu	90 min	Global increase in brain MRglu. Greatest increases in frontomedial, frontolateral, anterior cingulate, and temporomedial cortex. Smaller increases in the basal ganglia and sensorimotor and occipital cortices. Correlation of psychotomimetic symptoms with increases in prefrontal, anterior cingulate, and temporomedial cortices and putamen	Vollenweider et al. (1997)
PET/binding	7 Male healthy volunteers	Psilocybin (oral)	0.25 mg/kg	Randomized single-blind design. Binding of [^{11}C] raclopride to D2 receptors in striatum	Not clear: after 80 min and before 140 min	Decreased [^{11}C] raclopride receptor binding potential bilaterally in caudate and putamen, consistent with an increase in endogenous dopamine. Changes were correlated with depersonalization associated with euphoria	Vollenweider, Vontobel, Hell, and Leenders (1999)
PET/MRglu	8 Healthy volunteers	Psilocybin (oral)	0.2 mg/kg	Double-blind, placebo-controlled design; [^{18}F] FDG-assessed MRglu	110–120 min	Increased MRglu in different right hemispheric frontotemporal cortical regions, predominantly in anterior cingulate. Metabolic rates decreased in the thalamus. Attenuation of cognitive activation-related increases in left frontocortical regions	Gouzoulis-Mayfrank, Schreckenberger, et al. (1999) and Gouzoulis-Mayfrank, Thelen, et al. (1999)
EEG	50 Healthy volunteers	Psilocybin (oral)	0.17 or 0.215 mg/kg	Data from three different studies, all of them with a placebo-controlled fixed-order (placebo then psilocybin) double-blinded design	60 min	Decreased density of neuronal oscillations at 1.5–20 Hz within a neural network composed by the anterior cingulate cortex (ACC), posterior cingulate cortex (PCC), and parahippocampal regions. Intensity levels of psilocybin-induced spiritual experience and insightfulness correlated with lagged phase synchronization of delta oscillations (1.5–4 Hz) between the retrosplenial cortex, the parahippocampus, and the lateral orbitofrontal area	Kometer, Pokorny, Seifritz, and Volleinweider (2015)

MEG	15 Male healthy volunteers	Psilocybin (IV)	2 mg	Fixed-order (first placebo, then psilocybin) single-blinded design	Immediate	Spontaneous cortical oscillatory reduced by psilocybin in posterior association cortices from 1 to 50 Hz and from 8 to 100 Hz in frontal association cortices. Large decrease in the oscillatory power was observed in regions of the default mode network. No effect on low level visually induced and motor-induced gamma-band oscillations	Muthukumaraswamy et al. (2013)
fMRI/BOLD	10 Healthy volunteers	Psilocybin (IV)	2 mg	Volunteers submitted to drug and placebo separated by about 7 days	7½ min	Data acquisition during 16 s period while subjects imagined reexperiencing positive memories, after being exposed to visual cues for 6 s. Increased activity of visual and other sensory cortices during recollection. Stronger memory vividness and visual imagery. Significant correlation between subjective well-being at follow-up and memory vividness	Carhart-Harris, Leech, Williams, et al. (2012)
fMRI/ASL and BOLD	30 Healthy volunteers	Psilocybin (IV)	2 mg	Task-free placebo-controlled design; 15 volunteers for arterial spin-labeling perfusion and 15 for BOLD fMRI	Immediate	Only decreases in cerebral blood flow and BOLD signal were present. Decreases were more intense in thalamus, ACC, and PCC. Magnitude of decreased activity in ACC/medial prefrontal cortex (mPFC) predicted the intensity of the subjective effects. Connectivity analysis using medial prefrontal seed indicated significant decrease in positive coupling between mPFC and PCC	Carhart-Harris, Erritzoe, et al. (2012)
fMRI/BOLD	15 Healthy volunteers	Psilocybin (IV)	2 mg	Task-free placebo-controlled design	Immediate	Increased connectivity (ie, decreased orthogonality) between DMN and task-positive network. Different from sedation (where DMN–TPN orthogonality is also increased), decrease in thalamocortical functional connectivity was absent	Carhart-Harris et al. (2013)
						Wider repertoire of connectivity	Tagliazucchi, Carhart-Harris, Leech, Nutt, and Chialvo (2014)
						Higher connectivity defined by the appearance of several low stability transient structures and a few persistent structures	Petri et al. (2014)

Continued

Table 2 EEG and Imaging Studies with Psilocybin, Mescaline, and LSD—cont'd

Method	Subjects	Drug	Dosage	Design	Start of Acquisition After Dosing	Effects of Psychedelic Substance	References
				Comparison with a similar study using MDMA		Increased between-network RSFC with psilocybin and not MDMA. Decreased RSFC between visual and sensorimotor resting-state networks was also observed	Roseman, Leech, Feilding, Nutt, and Carhart-Harris (2014)
fMRI/BOLD	25 Healthy volunteers	Psilocybin (oral)	0.16 mg/kg	Double-blind crossover design; focus on the amygdala	70–90 min	Lower amygdala reactivity to negative and neutral stimuli. Correlation between psilocybin-induced attenuation of right amygdala reactivity in response to negative stimuli and psilocybin-induced increase in positive mood state	Kraehenmann et al. (2015)
fMRI/ASL and BOLD MEG	20 Healthy volunteers	LSD (IV)	75 μg	Placebo-controlled, within-subjects/crossover balanced-order design	ASL 100 min BOLD 135 min MEG 225 min	Increased visual cortex CBF, RSFC, and decreased alpha power, correlating with visual hallucinations; decreased DMN integrity, parahippocampus–retrosplenial cortex RSFC, and delta and alpha power (in the PCC), correlating with ego dissolution; decreased DMN activity	Carhart-Harris, Muthukumaraswamy, et al. (2016)

Note: *ASL*, arterial spin labeling; *ACC*, anterior cingulate cortex; *BOLD*, blood-oxygen-level-dependent contrast imaging; *CBF*, cerebral blood flow; *DMN*, default mode network; *EEG*, electroencephalography; *fMRI*, functional magnetic resonance imaging; *FDG*, fluorodesoxiglicose; *MEG*, magnetoencephalography; *MRglu*, glucose metabolic rate; *mPFC*, medial prefrontal cortex; *PET*, positron emission tomography; *PCC*, posterior cingulate cortex; *RSFC*, resting-state functional connectivity; *SPECT*, single-photon emission computed tomography; *TPN*, task-positive network.

Psilocybin decreased power (1.5–20 Hz) was observed within a neural network comprising the anterior and posterior cingulate cortices and the parahippocampal regions. Furthermore, the intensity of the psilocybin-induced spiritual experience correlated with the phase-lagged synchronization of delta oscillations between the retrosplenial cortex, the parahippocampus, and the lateral orbitofrontal area (Kometer et al., 2015). Psilocybin, D-methamphetamine, and 3,4-methylenedioxyethylamphetamine (MDE, an empathogen with properties similar to MDMA) were evaluated in healthy volunteers ($n=8$) in another double-blind, placebo-controlled ^{18}F FDG PET study. Psilocybin increased MRglu in various frontotemporal cortical regions, predominantly in the ACC, and mostly in the right hemisphere. Psilocybin-induced mental state was compared to acute psychosis, where frontal hyperreactivity is present at rest, but is also associated with a reduced capacity to recruit prefrontal regions upon cognitive demand (Gouzoulis-Mayfrank, Schreckenberger, et al., 1999; Gouzoulis-Mayfrank, Thelen, et al., 1999).

fMRI has also been used to study the acute effects of psilocybin. Ten healthy volunteers recalled positive autobiographical memories during two fMRI sessions under the influence of psilocybin (2 mg, intravenous), or placebo, separated by approximately 7 days. Psilocybin was associated with increased activity in visual cortices. Vividness of the memory and visual imagery was stronger with psilocybin. Furthermore, there was a significant correlation between subjective well-being at follow-up and vividness of the positive memory (Carhart-Harris, Leech, et al., 2012).

In another fMRI study, arterial spin labeling was used to evaluate CBF-related changes after intravenous administration of psilocybin (2 mg) or saline. Decreased activity in ACC/mPFC correlated with the intensity of subjective effects, as measured by a visual analog scale. Moreover, functional connectivity analysis revealed a significant decrease in positive coupling between the mPFC and the PCC (Carhart-Harris et al., 2013). In a follow-up study, different functional connectivity patterns were explored, suggesting that psilocybin increases brain connectivity overall when compared to placebo (Tagliazucchi et al., 2014). The psychedelic state is characterized by higher connectivity, defined by the appearance of several low stability, transient structures and a few persistent ones that were not observed with placebo (Petri et al., 2014). In a reanalysis of the same data, changes in resting-state functional connectivity (RSFC) between different resting-state networks (RSN) were measured. Data following exposure to psilocybin were compared to data following MDMA exposure. Psilocybin, but not MDMA, generally increased between RSFC networks (Roseman et al.,

2014). Decreased RSFC between visual and sensorimotor RSN was also observed. Thus, current evidence suggests that RSFC networks become less differentiated in the psychedelic state (eg, Muthukumaraswamy et al., 2013).

Amygdala reactivity to negative or neutral stimuli was lower following psilocybin than following placebo administration. A correlation was found between psilocybin-induced attenuation of the BOLD response in the right amygdala in response to negative stimuli and a psilocybin-induced increase in positive mood state (Kraehenmann et al., 2015, 2016). Such results indicate a positive effect of psilocybin on emotion processing, which suggests possible therapeutic properties.

2.3 Mescaline

Mescaline, isolated by Arthur Heffter in 1897, is the active component of psychedelic cacti such as peyote (*Lophophora williamsii*) and wachuma (*Echinopsis pachanoi*, also known as San Pedro). Similar to the other classic psychedelics, mescaline is a $5HT_{2A/2C}$ agonist and one of the most selectively serotonergic psychedelic (Ray, 2010). The usual dose of mescaline in humans is between 300 and 500 mg and its effects last for 6–8 h (Halberstadt, 2015; Shulgin, 1980). Twelve healthy, male volunteers, ingesting a dose of 500 mg of mescaline sulfate were compared to 12 age-matched male who were given placebo. After intake (4.5 h), subjects were scanned with ^{99m}Tc-HMPAO SPECT, and showed a pattern of hyperfrontality when compared to placebo (Hermle et al., 1992), which was correlated with psychotomimetic symptomatology (Hermle et al., 1998).

2.4 Lysergic Acid Diethylamide

LSD is psychoactive in very small amounts: effects are noticeable at about 25 μg, with typical doses between ~50 and 150 μg. Effects of LSD can last 8–14 h depending on the dose and tolerance due to repeated ingestion (Passie, Halpern, Stichtenoth, Emrich, & Hintzen, 2008; Shulgin, 1980). As seen in EEG studies of mescaline and psilocybin (eg, Loosemore & Harley, 2010; Monroe, Heath, Mickle, & Llewellyn, 1957), early EEG studies with LSD reported consistent findings including decreased broadband power and increased peak frequencies particularly in the frontal cortex (eg, Fink, 1969; Itil, 1968; Oughourlian, Rougeul, & Verdeaux, 1971). More recently, it was found that LSD has significant effects on the visual system, showing increased visual cortex CBF, decreased visual cortex alpha power, and a greatly expanded primary visual cortex (V1) functional connectivity profile. Moreover, likewise other psychedelics, LSD decreases the DMN connectivity (Carhart-Harris, Muthukumaraswamy, et al., 2016).

2.5 Summary of Current Brain Research in Psychedelics

Despite gaps in our current knowledge, occasional contradictory reports, and problems inherent to pharmacological research studies (eg, differentiating a brain response due to the direct action of the pharmaceutical agent from a "psychological" effect; consistency/standardization of substance preparation, dosing, administration, etc.; unique pharmacodynamics properties of each psychedelic compound), there are some consistent findings in the current psychedelic literature (please refer to Figs. 1 and 2). For example, EEG studies suggest that psychedelics induce a broad power reduction, most prominent in alpha and theta bands and increased peak frequency, especially for alpha (Dafters, Duffy, O'Donnell, & Bouquet, 1999; Hughes, 1996). SPECT/PET studies suggest that psychedelics increase CBF in key regions involved in emotional processing, such as the ACC and insula. A common finding in neuroimaging studies (eg, fMRI) is reduced activity in key hubs of the DMN, particularly of the PCC/precuneus (Carhart-Harris et al., 2013; Palhano-Fontes et al., 2015).

Another persistent finding is that psychedelics have pronounced effects on the visual system (Carhart-Harris, Muthukumaraswamy, et al., 2016; de Araujo et al., 2012). This area of investigation now requires a more refined description of the effects of psychedelics on the visual system since literature does not clearly differentiate true hallucinations, visual illusions, pseudohallucinations, or visual imagery facilitation. The valence of images and their integration with memories and affective states may be important in considering the therapeutic value of psychedelics.

3. PSYCHEDELICS AS THERAPEUTIC TOOLS

Psychedelics (eg, LSD, mescaline, psilocybin, DMT) were extensively explored as therapeutic tools before they became classified as illicit substances. Indeed, a rich literature focusing on the therapeutic potential of psychedelics, including treatment of depression, neurosis, obsessive–compulsive disorder, and addiction flourished in the 1950–1960s. The feeling of subjective wellness after the use of psychedelics, referred to as

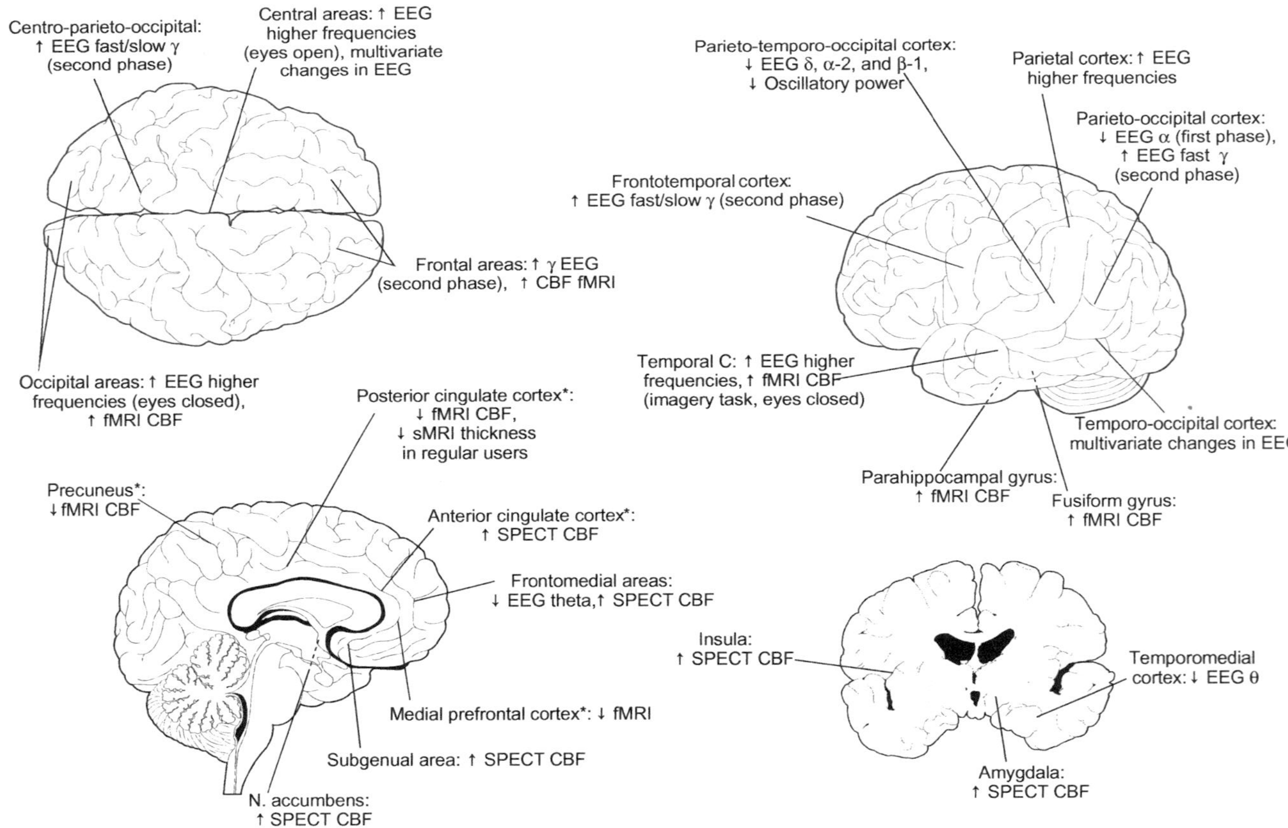

Fig. 1 Summary of results of EEG and imaging studies with ayahuasca: localized effects in the central nervous system. Default mode networks hubs are marked with an asterisk (*). *Note*: *CBF*, cerebral blood flow; *EEG*, electroencephalography; *fMRI*, functional magnetic resonance imaging; *MR*, metabolic rate; *MEG*, magnetoencephalography; *PET*, positron emission tomography; *psilo*, psilocybin; *PO*, per os; *IV*, intravenous; *RSFC*, resting-state functional connectivity.

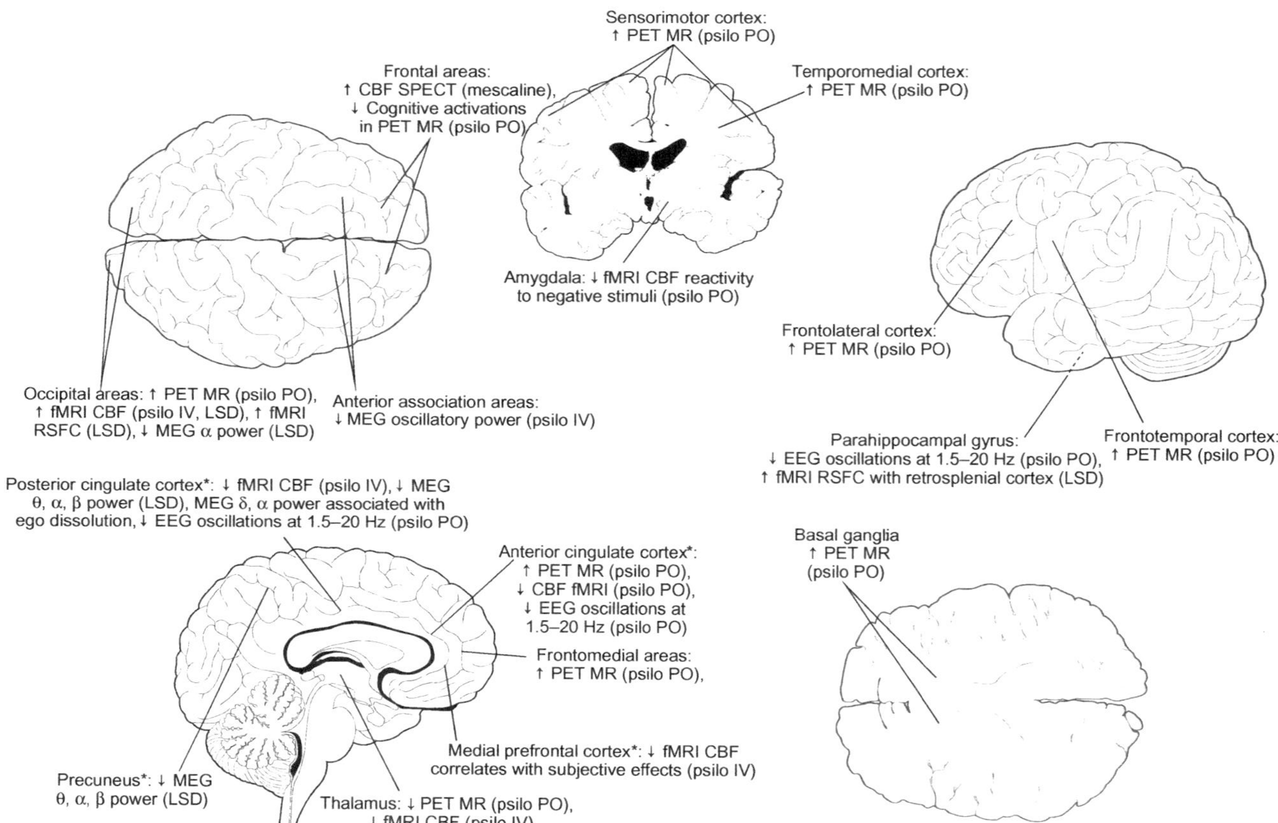

Fig. 2 Summary of results of EEG and imaging studies with psilocybin, mescaline, and LSD: localized effects in the central nervous system. Default mode networks hubs are marked with an asterisk (*). *Note*: *CBF*, cerebral blood flow; *EEG*, electroencephalography; *fMRI*, functional magnetic resonance imaging; *sMRI*, structural magnetic resonance imaging.

an "afterglow" (Majić, Schmidt, & Gallinat, 2015), has been reported in the literature since the 1960s (eg, Pahnke, 1969). In contrast to most antidepressants, psychedelics promote a positive mood almost immediately (Carhart-Harris, Bolstridge, et al., 2016; Osório et al., 2015; Sanches et al., 2016).

Early evaluation of psychedelics as chemical models of psychosis (ie, psychotomimetics or substances that induce states that mimic psychosis) suggested that at least some psychotic symptoms are induced by endogenous activations of $5HT_{2A}$ pathways, as observed using LSD in drug-discriminant animal studies. Such findings led to development of risperidone, an antipsychotic that in addition to blocking dopamine receptors, inhibits $5HT_{2A}$ receptors (Colpaert, 2003). Modern studies continue to use psychedelics as a source of insight into psychosis in general and schizophrenia in particular (Halberstadt & Geyer, 2013).

Treatment of both depression and addiction with psychedelics has shown promise. A growing literature indicates that psychedelics have antidepressant effects. Ayahuasca (Osório et al., 2015; Sanches et al., 2016) and psilocybin (Carhart-Harris, Bolstridge, et al., 2016) in open-label studies show potential antidepressant effects. As part of an ongoing investigation on the potential of ayahuasca to treat depressive states (Osório et al., 2015), a SPECT study was performed in 17 patients with recurrent depression 8 h after intake (Sanches et al., 2016). Ayahuasca, donated by Santo Daime, was administered *in natura* using an open-label design, and depression severity was assessed using the Hamilton Rating Scale for Depression (HAM-D) and the Montgomery–Åsberg Depression Rating Scale (MADRS). A significant decrease in ratings of depression was reported on both scales at 80 min after intake, a finding that persisted for 21 days. SPECT, performed 8 h after ayahuasca intake, showed significant CBF increases in the left nucleus accumbens, right insula, and left subgenual area. Similarly, two oral doses (10 and 25 mg) of psilocybin were given to 12 patients with moderate-to-severe treatment-resistant depression. Outcomes were measured with the quick inventory of depressive symptoms. Compared to baseline, depression symptoms were significantly reduced after 1 week and effects were sustained after 3 months after high-dose treatment (Carhart-Harris, Bolstridge, et al., 2016).

Based on results of early studies using LSD and other psychedelics, the scientific studies of ayahuasca in humans (Doering-Silveira et al., 2005; Fábregas et al., 2010; Grob et al., 1996), and anthropological and qualitative accounts from the ritual and religious use of psychedelics (Labate, Dos Santos, Anderson, Mercante, & Barbosa, 2014; Loizaga-Velder & Verres, 2014;

Mercante, 2013), a number of scientists began to explore the use of psychedelics for the treatment of drug-related disorders (eg, Bogenschutz & Johnson, 2016; Bogenschutz & Pommy, 2012; Brierley & Davidson, 2012; Dos Santos, Osório, Crippa, & Hallak, 2016; Frecska, Bokor, & Winkelman, 2016; Halpern, 1996, 2007; Liester & Prickett, 2012; Nunes et al., 2016; Ross, 2012; Winkelman, 2014). Indeed, a contemporary meta-analytic examination of early LSD studies found evidence for a beneficial effect of LSD on alcohol-use disorders (Krebs & Johansen, 2012). Results from modern observational and clinical trials are currently in a preliminary phase. Taken together, though, they are promising and seem to suggest a therapeutic effect of psychedelics on some psychiatric disease states.

In the seminal Project Hoasca, 15 male members of the UDV and 15 matched controls were given standardized questionnaires. Though the data were retrospective and the sample was small, the religious use of ayahuasca seemed to present a strong and positive impact in the lives of UDV members (Grob et al., 1996). UDV membership was also associated with reduced drug abuse in teenagers (Doering-Silveira et al., 2005). A survey of almost 1700 UDV members suggested lower rates of addiction relative to the general population (Barbosa, Tófoli, Bogenschutz, & Winkelman, 2014). Similarly, members of Santo Daime relative to the general population appear to have fewer psychiatric diagnoses of drug abuse (Fábregas et al., 2010). Therefore, although more studies are clearly necessary, current data seem to suggest that psychedelics have antiaddictive properties.

Additional studies have shown reduced addict-like behaviors in addicted patients who participated in an ayahuasca workshop with South American shamans (Thomas, Lucas, Capler, Tupper, & Martin, 2013). A study with mice demonstrated that ayahuasca inhibits the development of an animal model of alcohol dependence (Oliveira-Lima et al., 2015). Open-label study with psilocybin presented encouraging results for both alcohol and tobacco cessation: significant decreases in drinking behaviors were observed (Bogenschutz et al., 2015), and 80% of participating subjects achieved tobacco abstinence at 6-month follow-up (Johnson, Garcia-Romeu, Cosimano, & Griffiths, 2014).

4. POTENTIAL MECHANISMS OF PSYCHEDELIC TREATMENT EFFICACY

Functional activity of the DMN appears to be disrupted in a number of mental disorders, including addiction (Carhart-Harris & Nutt, 2013;

Chanraud, Pitel, Pfefferbaum, & Sullivan, 2011; Ma et al., 2011, 2015; Müller-Oehring, Jung, Pfefferbaum, Sullivan, & Schulte, 2015; Weiland, Sabbineni, Calhoun, Welsh, & Hutchison, 2015; Wetherill et al., 2015). These disruptions are complex and still not clearly elucidated, and it is too soon to suggest that the potential therapeutic role of psychedelics may come from their effect on the DMN. Such a mechanism would also seem contradictory based on findings that with the exception of alcohol, most addictive substances show reduced DMN connectivity and most psychedelics have also been shown to acutely reduce DMN connectivity.

In subjects with alcohol-use disorders relative to controls, DMN regions appear to be hyperconnected (Zhu, Cortes, Mathur, Tomasi, & Momenan, 2015; Zhu, Dutta, et al., 2015). Increased functional connectivity correlated with scores on an alcohol dependence scale. Alcohol-dependent subjects compared to controls also showed decreased functional connectivity of the precuneus after alcohol administration (Shokri-Kojori, Tomasi, Wiers, Wang, & Volkow, 2016). Considering such findings, alcoholism seems to be the most promising candidate for DMN studies investigating psychedelics for the treatment of addiction.

Another use of psychedelics in treatment is to increase interoception and self-awareness (DeWitt, Ketcherside, McQueeny, Dunlop, & Filbey, 2015), which may help in both psychiatric and addictive states. Mindfulness, likewise psychedelics, decreases activity of the DMN (Doll, Holzel, Boucard, Wohlschlager, & Sorg, 2015; King et al., 2016). Evaluation of the interaction between mindfulness techniques and psychedelic states may provide insights into better quality of life (Mackenzie, 2014; Soler et al., 2016).

Indirect activity of psychedelics on brain dopamine systems may be relevant to substance-use disorders (eg, Everitt, 2014; Kalivas, Volkow, & Seamans, 2005; Moeller, London, & Northoff, 2016; Volkow, Fowler, & Wang, 2003; Zou et al., 2015). For example, harmine and psilocin can increase dopamine in the ventral striatum/nucleus accumbens via $5HT_{2A/2C}$ receptor stimulation (Brierley & Davidson, 2013). LSD, psilocybin, and DMT may also effect dopamine transmission, though not necessarily in the nucleus accumbens. Imaging studies do not generally note a remarkable effect of psychedelics on the mesolimbic dopaminergic reward system. By contrast, a number of brain regions with an emerging role in the initiation or maintenance of addiction (eg, amygdala, hippocampus, insula, and medial prefrontal cortex) are directly influenced by psychedelics.

From a molecular perspective, available evidence suggests that psychedelics increase the expression of brain-derived neurotrophic factor

(BDNF) (Vollenweider & Kometer, 2010). BDNF increases are associated with the mitigation of symptoms of anxiety and depression: the increase in BDNF associated with use of antidepressants (eg, SSRI) coincides with the beginning of their therapeutic efficacy, typically 2 weeks after initiation (Bjorkholm & Monteggia, 2016). A more rapid effect of psychedelics may be associated with BDNF increases primarily in cortical pyramidal cells of layer V via a mechanism involving stimulation of $5HT_{2A}$ receptors (Vollenweider & Kometer, 2010).

Ayahuasca may additionally increase BDNF via at least one of the β-carbolines, namely, harmine, as demonstrated in animals. Indeed, β-carbolines may have independent antidepressant and anxiolytic properties possibly associated with direct stimulation of serotonin receptors or by MAO inhibition (Dos Santos et al., 2016). Similarly, THH can act as an SSRI and increase serotonin levels. Such hypotheses, however, fail to explain the apparently immediate antidepressant properties of ayahuasca.

DMT, in the few isolated studies in humans, seems to have antianxiety effects (Dos Santos et al., 2016). This is likely due to stimulation of serotonin $5HT_{2A}$ receptors. However, DMT is also a natural ligand for the sigma-1, intracellular chaperone receptor. Although the molecular roles of sigma-1 receptors remain to be explored, DMT has been identified as one of its natural and endogenous ligands (Fontanilla et al., 2009). Indeed, it has been hypothesized that dysfunction of sigma-1 receptors is associated with depression, anxiety, and substance-use-related disorders. A number of antidepressants have been shown to bind to sigma-1 receptors, and conversely, ligands of sigma-1 receptors have antidepressant effects in animal models of depression (Hayashi, Tsai, Mori, Fujimoto, & Su, 2011).

5. CLOSING REMARKS

There are many aspects of psychedelic consumption that may be beneficial beyond what may be adequately quantified in a laboratory setting (Garcia-Romeu, Griffiths, & Johnson, 2014; Griffiths, Richards, Johnson, McCann, & Jesse, 2008; MacLean, Johnson, & Griffiths, 2011). For example, traditional users of psychedelic plants often note the presence of a guiding instance, as well as visions that can be therapeutic as "didactic scenes" are common during ayahuasca use (eg, Shanon, 2003). Finally, psychedelic users often report spiritual experiences (eg, Barrett, Johnson, & Griffiths, 2015) and the ritual and religious use of peyote or ayahuasca is legal in many countries. Such considerations are not outside the scope of our modern attempts to treat addiction since after all, Alcoholics Anonymous, still one of the mainstays of treatment of alcoholism, includes a spiritual dimension. The goal then is not to deny, but to understand the spiritual/mystical components of psychedelics and provide research to assist therapists and other health professionals to exploit such properties of psychedelics to help those seeking relief from psychiatric symptoms or addiction. This is an open path for exploration with modern EEG and imaging techniques.

REFERENCES

Barbanoj, M. J., Riba, J., Clos, S., Gimenez, S., Grasa, E., & Romero, S. (2008). Daytime ayahuasca administration modulates REM and slow-wave sleep in healthy volunteers. *Psychopharmacology (Berl), 196*, 315–326.

Barbosa, P. C. R., Tófoli, L. F., Bogenschutz, M. P., & Winkelman, M. J. (2014). Assessment of alcohol use and dependence among religious users of hoasca. *Alcoholism: Clinical and Experimental Research, 38*(Suppl. 1), 144A.

Barrett, F. S., Johnson, M. W., & Griffiths, R. R. (2015). Validation of the revised mystical experience questionnaire in experimental sessions with psilocybin. *Journal of Psychopharmacology, 29*, 1182–1190.

Bjorkholm, C., & Monteggia, L. M. (2016). BDNF—A key transducer of antidepressant effects. *Neuropharmacology, 102*, 72–79.

Bogenschutz, M. P. (2013). Studying the effects of classic hallucinogens in the treatment of alcoholism: Rationale, methodology, and current research with psilocybin. *Current Drug Abuse Reviews, 6*, 17–29.

Bogenschutz, M. P., Forcehimes, A. A., Pommy, J. A., Wilcox, C. E., Barbosa, P. C., & Strassman, R. J. (2015). Psilocybin-assisted treatment for alcohol dependence: A proof-of-concept study. *Journal of Psychopharmacology, 29*, 289–299.

Bogenschutz, M. P., & Johnson, M. W. (2016). Classic hallucinogens in the treatment of addictions. *Progress in Neuro-Psychopharmacology & Biological Psychiatry, 64*, 250–258.

Bogenschutz, M. P., & Pommy, J. M. (2012). Therapeutic mechanisms of classic hallucinogens in the treatment of addictions: From indirect evidence to testable hypotheses. *Drug Testing and Analysis, 4*, 543–555.

Bouso, J. C., Palhano-Fontes, F., Rodríguez-Fornells, A., et al. (2015). Long-term use of psychedelic drugs is associated with differences in brain structure and personality in humans. *European Neuropsychopharmacology, 25*(4), 483–492. http://dx.doi.org/10.1016/j.euroneuro.2015.01.008.

Brierley, D. I., & Davidson, C. (2012). Developments in harmine pharmacology—Implications for ayahuasca use and drug-dependence treatment. *Progress in Neuro-Psychopharmacology & Biological Psychiatry, 39*, 263–272.

Brierley, D. I., & Davidson, C. (2013). Harmine augments electrically evoked dopamine efflux in the nucleus accumbens shell. *Journal of Psychopharmacology, 27*, 98–108.

Callaway, J. C., Raymon, L. P., Hearn, W. L., McKenna, D. J., Grob, C. S., Brito, G. S., et al. (1996). Quantitation of N,N-dimethyltryptamine and harmala alkaloids in human plasma after oral dosing with ayahuasca. *Journal of Analytical Toxicology, 20*, 492–497.

Carhart-Harris, R. L., Bolstridge, M., Rucker, J., Day, C. M., Erritzoe, D., Kaelen, M., et al. (2016). Psilocybin with psychological support for treatment-resistant depression: An open-label feasibility study. *The Lancet Psychiatry, 3*(7), 619–627.

Carhart-Harris, R. L., Erritzoe, D., Williams, T., Stone, J. M., Reed, L. J., Colasanti, A., et al. (2012). Neural correlates of the psychedelic state as determined by fMRI studies

with psilocybin. *Proceedings of the National Academy of Sciences of the United States of America, 109*, 2138–2143.
Carhart-Harris, R. L., Leech, R., Erritzoe, D., Williams, T. M., Stone, J. M., Evans, J., et al. (2013). Functional connectivity measures after psilocybin inform a novel hypothesis of early psychosis. *Schizophrenia Bulletin, 39*, 1343–1351.
Carhart-Harris, R. L., Leech, R., Williams, T. M., et al. (2012). Implications for psychedelic-assisted psychotherapy: Functional magnetic resonance imaging study with psilocybin. *The British Journal of Psychiatry, 200*(3), 238–244. http://dx.doi.org/10.1192/bjp.bp.111.103309.
Carhart-Harris, R. L., Muthukumaraswamy, S., Roseman, L., Kaelen, M., Droog, W., Murphy, K., et al. (2016). Neural correlates of the LSD experience revealed by multimodal neuroimaging. *Proceedings of the National Academy of Sciences of the United States of America, 113*, 4853–4858.
Carhart-Harris, R. L., & Nutt, D. J. (2013). Experienced drug users assess the relative harms and benefits of drugs: A web-based survey. *Journal of Psychoactive Drugs, 45*, 322–328.
Carhart-Harris, R. L., Williams, T. M., Sessa, B., Tyacke, R. J., Rich, A. S., Feilding, A., et al. (2011). The administration of psilocybin to healthy, hallucinogen-experienced volunteers in a mock-functional magnetic resonance imaging environment: A preliminary investigation of tolerability. *Journal of Psychopharmacology, 25*, 1562–1567.
Chanraud, S., Pitel, A. L., Pfefferbaum, A., & Sullivan, E. V. (2011). Disruption of functional connectivity of the default-mode network in alcoholism. *Cerebral Cortex, 21*, 2272–2281.
Colpaert, F. C. (2003). Discovering risperidone: The LSD model of psychopathology. *Nature Reviews. Drug Discovery, 2*, 315–320.
Dafters, R. I., Duffy, F., O'Donnell, P. J., & Bouquet, C. (1999). Level of use of 3,4-methylenedioxymethamphetamine (MDMA or Ecstasy) in humans correlates with EEG power and coherence. *Psychopharmacology (Berl), 145*, 82–90.
Dakwar, E., Levin, F., Foltin, R. W., Nunes, E. V., & Hart, C. L. (2014). The effects of subanesthetic ketamine infusions on motivation to quit and cue-induced craving in cocaine-dependent research volunteers. *Biological Psychiatry, 76*, 40–46.
de Araujo, D. B., Ribeiro, S., Cecchi, G. A., Carvalho, F. M., Sanchez, T. A., Pinto, J. P., et al. (2012). Seeing with the eyes shut: Neural basis of enhanced imagery following ayahuasca ingestion. *Human Brain Mapping, 33*, 2550–2560.
DeWitt, S. J., Ketcherside, A., McQueeny, T. M., Dunlop, J. P., & Filbey, F. M. (2015). The hyper-sentient addict: An exteroception model of addiction. *The American Journal of Drug and Alcohol Abuse, 41*, 374–381.
Doering-Silveira, E., Grob, C. S., de Rios, M. D., Lopez, E., Alonso, L. K., Tacla, C., et al. (2005). Report on psychoactive drug use among adolescents using ayahuasca within a religious context. *Journal of Psychoactive Drugs, 37*, 141–144.
Doll, A., Holzel, B. K., Boucard, C. C., Wohlschlager, A. M., & Sorg, C. (2015). Mindfulness is associated with intrinsic functional connectivity between default mode and salience networks. *Frontiers in Human Neuroscience, 9*, 461.
Don, N. S., McDonough, B. E., Moura, G., Warren, C. A., Kawanishi, K., Tomita, H., et al. (1998). Effects of ayahuasca on the human EEG. *Phytomedicine, 5*, 87–96.
Dos Santos, R. G., Osório, F. L., Crippa, J. A., & Hallak, J. E. (2016). Antidepressive and anxiolytic effects of ayahuasca: A systematic literature review of animal and human studies. *Revista Brasileira de Psiquiatria, 38*, 65–72.
Dyck, E. (2009). Prairies, psychedelics and place: The dynamics of region in psychiatric research. *Health & Place, 15*, 888–894.
Everitt, B. J. (2014). Neural and psychological mechanisms underlying compulsive drug seeking habits and drug memories—Indications for novel treatments of addiction. *The European Journal of Neuroscience, 40*, 2163–2182.

Fábregas, J. M., González, D., Fondevila, S., Cutchet, M., Fernández, X., Barbosa, P. C., et al. (2010). Assessment of addiction severity among ritual users of ayahuasca. *Drug and Alcohol Dependence*, *111*, 257–261.

Fink, M. (1969). EEG and human psychopharmacology. *Annual Review of Pharmacology*, *9*, 241–258.

Fontanilla, D., Johannessen, M., Hajipour, A. R., Cozzi, N. V., Jackson, M. B., & Ruoho, A. E. (2009). The hallucinogen N,N-dimethyltryptamine (DMT) is an endogenous sigma-1 receptor regulator. *Science*, *323*, 934–937.

Frecska, E., Bokor, P., & Winkelman, M. (2016). The therapeutic potentials of ayahuasca: Possible effects against various diseases of civilization. *Frontiers in Pharmacology*, *7*, 35.

Garcia-Romeu, A., Griffiths, R. R., & Johnson, M. W. (2014). Psilocybin-occasioned mystical experiences in the treatment of tobacco addiction. *Current Drug Abuse Reviews*, *7*, 157–164.

Gasser, P., Holstein, D., Michel, Y., Doblin, R., Yazar-Klosinski, B., Passie, T., et al. (2014). Safety and efficacy of lysergic acid diethylamide-assisted psychotherapy for anxiety associated with life-threatening diseases. *The Journal of Nervous and Mental Disease*, *202*, 513–520.

Gouzoulis-Mayfrank, E., Schreckenberger, M., Sabri, O., Arning, C., Thelen, B., Spitzer, M., et al. (1999). Neurometabolic effects of psilocybin, 3,4-methylenedioxyethylamphetamine (MDE) and D-methamphetamine in healthy volunteers. A double-blind, placebo-controlled PET study with [^{18}F]FDG. *Neuropsychopharmacology*, *20*, 565–581.

Gouzoulis-Mayfrank, E., Thelen, B., Habermeyer, E., Kunert, H. J., Kovar, K. A., Lindenblatt, H., et al. (1999). Psychopathological, neuroendocrine and autonomic effects of 3,4-methylenedioxyethylamphetamine (MDE), psilocybin and D-methamphetamine in healthy volunteers. Results of an experimental double-blind placebo-controlled study. *Psychopharmacology (Berl)*, *142*, 41–50.

Griffiths, R., Richards, W., Johnson, M., McCann, U., & Jesse, R. (2008). Mystical-type experiences occasioned by psilocybin mediate the attribution of personal meaning and spiritual significance 14 months later. *Journal of Psychopharmacology*, *22*, 621–632.

Grob, C. S., McKenna, D. J., Callaway, J. C., Brito, G. S., Neves, E. S., Oberlaender, G., et al. (1996). Human psychopharmacology of hoasca, a plant hallucinogen used in ritual context in Brazil. *The Journal of Nervous and Mental Disease*, *184*, 86–94.

Halberstadt, A. L. (2015). Recent advances in the neuropsychopharmacology of serotonergic hallucinogens. *Behavioural Brain Research*, *277*, 99–120.

Halberstadt, A. L., & Geyer, M. A. (2013). Serotonergic hallucinogens as translational models relevant to schizophrenia. *The International Journal of Neuropsychopharmacology*, *16*, 2165–2180.

Halpern, J. H. (1996). The use of hallucinogens in the treatment of addiction. *Addiction Research*, *4*, 177–189.

Halpern, J. H. (2007). Hallucinogens in the treatment of alcoholism and other addictions. In M. J. Winkelman & T. B. Roberts (Eds.), *Psychedelic medicine: New evidence for psychedelics substances as treatments* (pp. 1–14). Westport, CT: Praeger Security International.

Hamilton, J. P., Farmer, M., Fogelman, P., & Gotlib, I. H. (2015). Depressive rumination, the default-mode network, and the dark matter of clinical neuroscience. *Biological Psychiatry*, *78*, 224–230.

Hasler, F., Bourquin, D., Brenneisen, R., Bar, T., & Vollenweider, F. X. (1997). Determination of psilocin and 4-hydroxyindole-3-acetic acid in plasma by HPLC-ECD and pharmacokinetic profiles of oral and intravenous psilocybin in man. *Pharmaceutica Acta Helvetiae*, *72*, 175–184.

Hayashi, T., Tsai, S. Y., Mori, T., Fujimoto, M., & Su, T. P. (2011). Targeting ligand-operated chaperone sigma-1 receptors in the treatment of neuropsychiatric disorders. *Expert Opinion on Therapeutic Targets*, *15*, 557–577.

Hermle, L., Funfgeld, M., Oepen, G., Botsch, H., Borchardt, D., Gouzoulis, E., et al. (1992). Mescaline-induced psychopathological, neuropsychological, and neurometabolic effects in normal subjects: Experimental psychosis as a tool for psychiatric research. *Biological Psychiatry*, *32*, 976–991.

Hermle, L., Gouzoulis-Mayfrank, E., & Spitzer, M. (1998). Blood flow and cerebral laterality in the mescaline model of psychosis. *Pharmacopsychiatry*, *31*(Suppl. 2), 85–91.

Hoffman, E., Hesselink, J. M. K., & Silveira-Barbosa, Y. W. M. (2001). Effects of a psychedelic, tropical tea, ayahuasca, on the electroencephalographic (EEG) activity of the human brain during a shamanistic ritual. *MAPS Bulletin*, *11*, 25–30.

Hughes, J. R. (1996). A review of the usefulness of the standard EEG in psychiatry. *Clinical Electroencephalography*, *27*, 35–39.

Itil, T. M. (1968). Electroencephalography and pharmacopsychiatry. In F. A. Freyhan, N. Pertrolowitsch, & P. E. Pichot (Eds.), *Clinical psychopharmacology: Modern problems of pharmacopsychiatry* (pp. 163–194). New York: Karger.

Johnson, M. W., Garcia-Romeu, A., Cosimano, M. P., & Griffiths, R. R. (2014). Pilot study of the 5-HT2AR agonist psilocybin in the treatment of tobacco addiction. *Journal of Psychopharmacology*, *28*, 983–992.

Kalivas, P. W., Volkow, N., & Seamans, J. (2005). Unmanageable motivation in addiction: A pathology in prefrontal-accumbens glutamate transmission. *Neuron*, *45*, 647–650.

King, A. P., Block, S. R., Sripada, R. K., Rauch, S., Giardino, N., Favorite, T., et al. (2016). Altered default mode network (DMN) resting state functional connectivity following a mindfulness-based exposure therapy for posttraumatic stress disorder (PTSD) in combat veterans of Afghanistan and Iraq. *Depression and Anxiety*, *33*, 289–299.

Kometer, M., Pokorny, T., Seifritz, E., & Volleinweider, F. X. (2015). Psilocybin-induced spiritual experiences and insightfulness are associated with synchronization of neuronal oscillations. *Psychopharmacology (Berl)*, *232*, 3663–3676.

Kometer, M., Schmidt, A., Jancke, L., & Vollenweider, F. X. (2013). Activation of serotonin 2A receptors underlies the psilocybin-induced effects on alpha oscillations, N170 visual-evoked potentials, and visual hallucinations. *The Journal of Neuroscience*, *33*, 10544–10551.

Kraehenmann, R., Preller, K. H., Scheidegger, M., Pokorny, T., Bosch, O. G., Seifritz, E., et al. (2015). Psilocybin-induced decrease in amygdala reactivity correlates with enhanced positive mood in healthy volunteers. *Biological Psychiatry*, *78*, 572–581.

Kraehenmann, R., Schmidt, A., Friston, K., Preller, K. H., Seifritz, E., & Vollenweider, F. X. (2016). The mixed serotonin receptor agonist psilocybin reduces threat-induced modulation of amygdala connectivity. *Neuroimage: Clinical*, *11*, 53–60.

Krebs, T. S., & Johansen, P. O. (2012). Lysergic acid diethylamide (LSD) for alcoholism: Meta-analysis of randomized controlled trials. *Journal of Psychopharmacology*, *26*, 994–1002.

Labate, B. C., & Cavnar, C. (2011). The expansion of the field of research on ayahuasca: Some reflections about the ayahuasca track at the 2010 MAPS "Psychedelic Science in the 21st Century" conference. *The International Journal on Drug Policy*, *22*, 174–178.

Labate, B. C., Dos Santos, R. G., Anderson, B. T., Mercante, M. S., & Barbosa, P. C. (2014). The treatment and handling of substance dependence with ayahuasca: Reflections on current and future research. In B. C. Labate & E. MacRae (Eds.), *Ayahuasca, ritual and religion in Brazil* (pp. 205–227). New York: Routledge.

Liester, M. B., & Prickett, J. I. (2012). Hypotheses regarding the mechanisms of ayahuasca in the treatment of addictions. *Journal of Psychoactive Drugs*, *44*, 200–208.

Loizaga-Velder, A., & Verres, R. (2014). Therapeutic effects of ritual ayahuasca use in the treatment of substance dependence—Qualitative results. *Journal of Psychoactive Drugs*, *46*, 63–72.

Loosemore, A., & Harley, T. (2010). *Brains and minds: On the usefulness of localization data to cognitive psychology*. Cambridge, MA: MIT Press.

Ma, N., Liu, Y., Fu, X. M., Li, N., Wang, C. X., Zhang, H., et al. (2011). Abnormal brain default-mode network functional connectivity in drug addicts. *PloS One, 6*, e16560.

Ma, X., Qiu, Y., Tian, J., Wang, J., Li, S., Zhan, W., et al. (2015). Aberrant default-mode functional and structural connectivity in heroin-dependent individuals. *PloS One, 10*, e0120861.

Mackenzie, R. (2014). What can neuroscience tell us about the potential of psychedelics in healthcare? How the neurophenomenology of psychedelics research could help us to flourish throughout our lives, as well as to enhance our dying. *Current Drug Abuse Reviews*, 7, 136–145.

MacLean, K. A., Johnson, M. W., & Griffiths, R. R. (2011). Mystical experiences occasioned by the hallucinogen psilocybin lead to increases in the personality domain of openness. *Journal of Psychopharmacology, 25*, 1453–1461.

Majić, T., Schmidt, T. T., & Gallinat, J. (2015). Peak experiences and the afterglow phenomenon: When and how do therapeutic effects of hallucinogens depend on psychedelic experiences? *Journal of Psychopharmacology, 29*, 241–253.

Mangini, M. (1998). Treatment of alcoholism using psychedelic drugs: A review of the program of research. *Journal of Psychoactive Drugs, 30*, 381–418.

McKenna, D. J. (2004). Clinical investigations of the therapeutic potential of ayahuasca: Rationale and regulatory challenges. *Pharmacology & Therapeutics, 102*, 111–129.

Mercante, M. S. (2013). Ayahuasca and the treatment of drug dependence. *Mana, 19*, 529–558.

Moeller, S. J., London, E. D., & Northoff, G. (2016). Neuroimaging markers of glutamatergic and GABAergic systems in drug addiction: Relationships to resting-state functional connectivity. *Neuroscience and Biobehavioral Reviews, 61*, 35–52.

Monroe, R. R., Heath, R. G., Mickle, W. A., & Llewellyn, R. C. (1957). Correlation of rhinencephalic electrograms with behavior; a study on humans under the influence of LSD and mescaline. *Electroencephalography and Clinical Neurophysiology, 9*, 623–642.

Müller-Oehring, E. M., Jung, Y. C., Pfefferbaum, A., Sullivan, E. V., & Schulte, T. (2015). The resting brain of alcoholics. *Cerebral Cortex, 25*, 4155–4168.

Muthukumaraswamy, S. D., Carhart-Harris, R. L., Moran, R. J., Brookes, M. J., Williams, T. M., Errtizoe, D., et al. (2013). Broadband cortical desynchronization underlies the human psychedelic state. *The Journal of Neuroscience, 33*, 15171–15183.

Naranjo, C. (1987). Ayahuasca imagery and the therapeutic property of the harmala alkaloids. *Journal of Mental Imagery, 11*, 131–136.

Nichols, D. E. (2004). Hallucinogens. *Pharmacology & Therapeutics, 101*, 131–181.

Nunes, A. A., Dos Santos, R. G., Osório, F. L., Sanches, R. F., Crippa, J. A., & Hallak, J. E. (2016). Effects of ayahuasca and its alkaloids on drug dependence: A systematic literature review of quantitative studies in animals and humans. *Journal of Psychoactive Drugs, 48*, 195–205.

Oliveira-Lima, A. J., Santos, R., Hollais, A. W., Gerardi-Junior, C. A., Baldaia, M. A., Wuo-Silva, R., et al. (2015). Effects of ayahuasca on the development of ethanol-induced behavioral sensitization and on a post-sensitization treatment in mice. *Physiology & Behavior, 142*, 28–36.

Oram, M. (2014). Efficacy and enlightenment: LSD psychotherapy and the Drug Amendments of 1962. *Journal of the History of Medicine and Allied Sciences, 69*, 221–250.

Osório, F. L., Sanches, R. F., Macedo, L. R., Dos Santos, R. G., Maia-de-Oliveira, J. P., Wichert-Ana, L., et al. (2015). Antidepressant effects of a single dose of ayahuasca in patients with recurrent depression: A preliminary report. *Revista Brasileira de Psiquiatria, 37*, 13–20.

Ott, J. (1994). *Ayahuasca analogues pangean entheogens*. Kennewick, WA: Natural Products Co.

Oughourlian, J. M., Rougeul, A., & Verdeaux, J. (1971). Action of hallucinogens on electroencephalograms. *Thérapie, 26*, 953–968.

Pahnke, W. N. (1969). Psychedelic drugs and mystical experience. *International Psychiatry Clinics, 5*, 149–162.

Palhano-Fontes, F., Andrade, K. C., Tófoli, L. F., Santos, A. C., Crippa, J. A., Hallak, J. E., et al. (2015). The psychedelic state induced by ayahuasca modulates the activity and connectivity of the default mode network. *PloS One, 10*, e0118143.

Passie, T., Halpern, J. H., Stichtenoth, D. O., Emrich, H. M., & Hintzen, A. (2008). The pharmacology of lysergic acid diethylamide: A review. *CNS Neuroscience & Therapeutics, 14*, 295–314.

Passie, T., Seifert, J., Schneider, U., & Emrich, H. M. (2002). The pharmacology of psilocybin. *Addiction Biology, 7*, 357–364.

Petri, G., Expert, P., Turkheimer, F., Carhart-Harris, R., Nutt, D., Hellyer, P. J., et al. (2014). Homological scaffolds of brain functional networks. *Journal of the Royal Society, Interface, 11*, 20140873.

Popik, P., Layer, R. T., & Skolnick, P. (1995). 100 Years of ibogaine: Neurochemical and pharmacological actions of a putative anti-addictive drug. *Pharmacological Reviews, 47*, 235–253.

Ray, T. S. (2010). Psychedelics and the human receptorome. *PloS One, 5*, e9019.

Riba, J., Anderer, P., Jane, F., Saletu, B., & Barbanoj, M. J. (2004). Effects of the South American psychoactive beverage ayahuasca on regional brain electrical activity in humans: A functional neuroimaging study using low-resolution electromagnetic tomography. *Neuropsychobiology, 50*, 89–101.

Riba, J., Anderer, P., Morte, A., Urbano, G., Jane, F., Saletu, B., et al. (2002). Topographic pharmaco-EEG mapping of the effects of the South American psychoactive beverage ayahuasca in healthy volunteers. *British Journal of Clinical Pharmacology, 53*, 613–628.

Riba, J., Romero, S., Grasa, E., Mena, E., Carrio, I., & Barbanoj, M. J. (2006). Increased frontal and paralimbic activation following ayahuasca, the pan-Amazonian inebriant. *Psychopharmacology (Berl), 186*, 93–98.

Riba, J., Valle, M., Urbano, G., Yritia, M., Morte, A., & Barbanoj, M. J. (2003). Human pharmacology of ayahuasca: Subjective and cardiovascular effects, monoamine metabolite excretion, and pharmacokinetics. *The Journal of Pharmacology and Experimental Therapeutics, 306*, 73–83.

Roseman, L., Leech, R., Feilding, A., Nutt, D. J., & Carhart-Harris, R. L. (2014). The effects of psilocybin and MDMA on between-network resting state functional connectivity in healthy volunteers. *Frontiers in Human Neuroscience, 8*, 204.

Ross, S. (2012). Serotonergic hallucinogens and emerging targets for addiction pharmacotherapies. *The Psychiatric Clinics of North America, 35*, 357–374.

Rowe, T. C. (2006). *Federal narcotics laws and the war on drugs: Money down a rat hole.* New York: Routledge.

Sanches, R. F., Osório, F. L., Dos Santos, R. G., Macedo, L. R., Maia-de-Oliveira, J. P., Wichert-Ana, L., et al. (2016). Antidepressant effects of a single dose of ayahuasca in patients with recurrent depression: A SPECT Study. *Journal of Clinical Psychopharmacology, 36*, 77–81.

Schenberg, E. E., Alexandre, J. F., Filev, R., Cravo, A. M., Sato, J. R., Muthukumaraswamy, S. D., et al. (2015). Acute biphasic effects of ayahuasca. *PloS One, 10*, e0137202.

Schultes, R. E. (1979). Hallucinogenic plants: Their earliest botanical descriptions. *Journal of Psychedelic Drugs, 11*, 13–24.

Sessa, B. (2012). *The psychedelic renaissance: Reassessing the role of psychedelic drugs in 21st century psychiatry and society.* London: Muswell Hill Press.

Sewell, R. A., Halpern, J. H., & Pope, H. G., Jr. (2006). Response of cluster headache to psilocybin and LSD. *Neurology, 66*, 1920–1922.

Shanon, B. (2003). *The antipodes of the mind: Charting the phenomenology of the ayahuasca experience* (1st ed.). New York: Oxford University Press Inc.
Shmulewitz, D., Greene, E. R., & Hasin, D. (2015). Commonalities and differences across substance use disorders: Phenomenological and epidemiological aspects. *Alcoholism, Clinical and Experimental Research, 39*, 1878–1900.
Shokri-Kojori, E., Tomasi, D., Wiers, C. E., Wang, G. J., & Volkow, N. D. (2016). Alcohol affects brain functional connectivity and its coupling with behavior: Greater effects in male heavy drinkers. *Molecular Psychiatry*. http://dx.doi.org/10.1038/mp.2016.25. (Epub ahead of print).
Shulgin, A. T. (1980). Profiles of psychedelic drugs. *Journal of Psychedelic Drugs, 12*, 173–174.
Soler, J., Elices, M., Franquesa, A., Barker, S., Friedlander, P., Feilding, A., et al. (2016). Exploring the therapeutic potential of ayahuasca: Acute intake increases mindfulness-related capacities. *Psychopharmacology, 233*, 823–829.
Stafford, P. (1992). *Psychedelics encyclopedia*. Berkeley, CA: Ronin Publishing, Inc.
Szabó, A., Kazai, A., Frecska, E., & Brys, Z. (2015). Psychedelics and quasi-psychedelics in the light of contemporary research: Medical cannabis, MDMA, salvinorin A, ibogaine and ayahuasca. *Neuropsychopharmacologia Hungarica, 17*, 120–128.
Tagliazucchi, E., Carhart-Harris, R., Leech, R., Nutt, D., & Chialvo, D. R. (2014). Enhanced repertoire of brain dynamical states during the psychedelic experience. *Human Brain Mapping, 35*, 5442–5456.
Thomas, G., Lucas, P., Capler, N. R., Tupper, K. W., & Martin, G. (2013). Ayahuasca-assisted therapy for addiction: Results from a preliminary observational study in Canada. *Current Drug Abuse Reviews, 6*, 30–42.
Tops, M., Boksem, M. A., Quirin, M., IJzerman, H., & Koole, S. L. (2014). Internally directed cognition and mindfulness: An integrative perspective derived from predictive and reactive control systems theory. *Frontiers in Psychology, 5*, 429.
Tylš, F., Páleníček, T., & Horáček, J. (2014). Psilocybin—Summary of knowledge and new perspectives. *European Neuropsychopharmacology, 24*, 342–356.
Volkow, N. D., Fowler, J. S., & Wang, G. J. (2003). The addicted human brain: Insights from imaging studies. *The Journal of Clinical Investigation, 111*, 1444–1451.
Vollenweider, F. X., & Kometer, M. (2010). The neurobiology of psychedelic drugs: Implications for the treatment of mood disorders. *Nature Reviews. Neuroscience, 11*, 642–651.
Vollenweider, F. X., Leenders, K. L., Scharfetter, C., Maguire, P., Stadelmann, O., & Angst, J. (1997). Positron emission tomography and fluorodeoxyglucose studies of metabolic hyperfrontality and psychopathology in the psilocybin model of psychosis. *Neuropsychopharmacology, 16*, 357–372.
Vollenweider, F. X., Vontobel, P., Hell, D., & Leenders, K. L. (1999). 5-HT modulation of dopamine release in basal ganglia in psilocybin-induced psychosis in man—A PET study with [11C]raclopride. *Neuropsychopharmacology, 20*(5), 424–433. http://dx.doi.org/10.1016/S0893-133X(98)00108-0.
Weiland, B. J., Sabbineni, A., Calhoun, V. D., Welsh, R. C., & Hutchison, K. E. (2015). Reduced executive and default network functional connectivity in cigarette smokers. *Human Brain Mapping, 36*, 872–882.
Wetherill, R. R., Fang, Z., Jagannathan, K., Childress, A. R., Rao, H., & Franklin, T. R. (2015). Cannabis, cigarettes, and their co-occurring use: Disentangling differences in default mode network functional connectivity. *Drug and Alcohol Dependence, 153*, 116–123.
Winkelman, M. (2014). Psychedelics as medicines for substance abuse rehabilitation: Evaluating treatments with LSD, peyote, ibogaine and ayahuasca. *Current Drug Abuse Reviews, 7*, 101–116.

Zhu, X., Cortes, C. R., Mathur, K., Tomasi, D., & Momenan, R. (2015). Model-free functional connectivity and impulsivity correlates of alcohol dependence: A resting-state study. *Addiction Biology*. http://dx.doi.org/10.1111/adb.12272. (Epub ahead of print).
Zhu, X., Dutta, N., Helton, S. G., Schwandt, M., Yan, J., Hodgkinson, C. A., et al. (2015). Resting-state functional connectivity and presynaptic monoamine signaling in alcohol dependence. *Human Brain Mapping*, *36*, 4808–4818.
Zou, F., Wu, X., Zhai, T., Lei, Y., Shao, Y., Jin, X., et al. (2015). Abnormal resting-state functional connectivity of the nucleus accumbens in multi-year abstinent heroin addicts. *Journal of Neuroscience Research*, *93*, 1693–1702.

INDEX

Note: Page numbers followed by "*f*" indicate figures, and "*t*" indicate tables.

I

K

L

M

N

O

P

CONTENTS OF RECENT VOLUMES

Volume 39

Volume 40

Volume 41

Volume 42

Volume 43

Volume 44

Volume 45

Volume 46

Volume 47

Volume 48

Volume 49

Volume 50

Volume 51

Volume 52

Volume 53

Volume 54

Volume 55

Volume 56

Volume 57

Volume 58

Volume 59

Volume 60

Volume 61

Volume 62

Volume 63

Volume 64

Volume 65

Volume 66

Volume 67

Volume 68

Volume 69

Volume 70

Volume 71

Volume 72

Volume 73

Volume 74

Volume 75

Volume 76

Volume 77

Volume 78

Volume 79

Volume 80

Volume 81

Volume 82

Volume 83

Volume 84

Volume 85

Volume 86

Volume 87

Volume 88

Volume 89

Volume 90

Volume 91

Volume 92

Volume 93

Volume 94

Volume 95

Volume 96

Volume 97

Volume 98

Volume 99

Volume 100

Volume 101

Volume 102

Volume 103

Volume 104

Volume 105

Volume 106

Volume 107

Volume 108

Volume 109

Volume 110

Volume 111

Volume 112

Volume 113

Volume 114

Volume 115

Volume 116

Volume 117

Volume 118

Volume 119

Volume 120

Volume 121

Volume 122

Volume 123

Volume 124

Volume 125

Volume 126

Volume 127

Volume 128

FSC
www.fsc.org
MIX
Papier | Fördert gute Waldnutzung
FSC® C083411

Kolibri 360 GmbH
Ferdinand-Jühlke-Straße 7
99095 Erfurt, Deutschland
produktsicherheit@kolibri360.de